Chest Imaging

Les R. Folio

Chest Imaging

An Algorithmic Approach to Learning

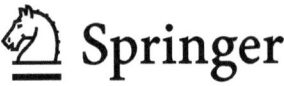
Springer

Les R. Folio, DO, MPH, FAOCR
Col (ret), USAF, MC, SFS
Clinical Associate Professor of Radiology
Philadelphia College of Osteopathic
Medicine
Philadelphia, PA
USA
lesfoli@pcom.edu

ISBN 978-1-4614-1316-5   e-ISBN 978-1-4614-1317-2
DOI 10.1007/978-1-4614-1317-2
Springer New York Dordrecht Heidelberg London

Library of Congress Control Number: 2011937481

Printed on acid-free paper

Springer is part of Springer Science+Business Media (www.springer.com)

*To the medical students, residents
and fellows I have taught chest imaging
over the years.*

Foreword

I was distinctly honored when Col (ret) Folio asked me to write this foreword, as he taught chest imaging throughout my student tenure at the Uniformed Services University (USU) in Bethesda, MD. He led the second year radiology lecture series for our class, to include the memorable CXR final oral exam event, and ran the fourth year radiology elective for several years, providing all the chest imaging presentations for hundreds of students. My fellow students and I found his pedagogical teaching techniques and course materials, such as RoboChest, useful in that he taught in a way one remembers, from findings to differential. This book reflects his teachings by breaking the chest x-ray into manageable components that the student of radiology can reasonably master in a short period of time.

The following text presents a unique approach to the CXR that includes mnemonics on most everything from the search pattern and diagnostic approach to disease processes that are retained for years. By reading this book, one can understand the complexity of interstitial disease (for example) with clever algorithms built in Excel® that provide a general understanding of an otherwise daunting and seemingly unlimited differential. And who could possibly forget the findings of hydropneumothorax with his balloon and milk in the glass analogy? Or the tram tracks in bronchiectasis from his straw in the sponge model? This text allows these teaching pearls to be shared for years to come.

The online directory structure of lung patterns on his www.robochest.com is unparalleled. When looking for the information needed, this website naturally guides the student of radiology in an interactive outline format that expands when more detail is desired. One always knows where they are on the pathway with breadcrumb trails, and can backtrack in a methodical fashion to get to a differential diagnosis. This basic launching platform to chest imaging is timeless and especially useful for many of us that will deploy with minimal resources in austere environments such as combat. This book contains everything RoboChest has, with many improvements, including clearer descriptions, annotations, and relations to the analogous models.

I am confident I will be reading this book several times over in the next few years, and I expect that when I deploy, it will be packed safely in my gear bag to take with me to help provide good medicine in combat situations. I believe I can speak for our entire graduating class: that no other teacher comes to mind when reading a CXR; he is a legend in our book. I hope you find this text and his teaching methods as useful as we did, and are fortunate enough to benefit from his inspiring lectures in the future.

– Captain "JD" Hoskins, President,
USU School of Medicine Class of 2011

Preface

This book is written for the "student of radiology" which historically has included medical students and radiology residents. Due to recent increased diversity in the medical team, I consider nurse practitioners, physician's assistants, nurses, medical students and radiology technicians to be included as students of radiology. The audience also includes residents and fellows of all clinical disciplines, especially ICU staff. The morning CXR review and rounds that follow (ICU, surgery, ID, etc.) are the pulse of any hospital. Even in combat hospitals the day starts with the CXR rounds, followed by ICU and other specialty rounds (surgery, infectious disease, etc.).

I am often asked how I came up with the RoboChest title for the first edition and the online content. It is very simple; the program we used to make the online version is called RoboHelp by Adobe®. With Adobe's® permission, I borrowed the "Robo" and added chest. It was designed to be help pages for a larger project that is still under development. These are the familiar help boxes that accompany popular programs that are organized in folders that can be opened for more detail.

In this edition, I have distilled the content of the search pattern to a very easy to remember mnemonic (ABCDS)×2 covering all aspects of the CXR.

The second mnemonic that helps guide the student of radiology through the diagnostic process is ID CD, or Identify, Define, Categorize, Differential. Using these and several other mnemonics introduced throughout the book, a beginner can build confidence reading CXRs.

The prior two versions of RoboChest book were meant as a guide to the launching website www.robochest.com. Although this book follows the same methodical pattern-driven approach to the chest x-ray, it is meant as a stand-alone introduction to chest imaging, while being augmented by the RoboChest website as a teaching tool. I hope you find this book as a valuable guide through the world of chest x-rays.

Les R. Folio, DO, MPH, FAOCR
Col (ret), USAF, MC, SFS

Educational Support and Funding

The original project "ChestWeb" was supported in part by the Henry M. Jackson Foundation (HMJF) and a Corporate Research and Development Award (CRADA) with Expert-24, USU, and HMJF. In addition, several intramural grants such as the USUS Dean's Endowment fund helped develop this teaching tool.

First printing: "RoboChest" v2.0: 15 Aug 2009

Second printing "RoboChest" v2.1: 15 Jul 2010

Acknowledgments

This product was initially created as a browser-based tool by the Education and Technology (ETI) Support Office at Uniformed Services University. After methodically organizing our lecture materials and other content into sections that would illuminate the complex art of the CXR, the ETI team developed the pages and the directory structure. The ETI Support Office is operated by Concurrent Technologies Corporation.

I would like to acknowledge Sofia Echelmeyer for her excellent artwork in several of the chapters. I would especially like to thank Dr. David Feigin of Johns Hopkins University for content based on his systematic teaching methods in the analysis of pulmonary patterns. I can safely say that Dr. Feigin taught me how to teach medical students chest x-ray.

Contents

Chapter 1
Introduction, Development
of the Algorithm, RoboChest
Introduction, Additional Tools

The Chest X-Ray (CXR, or chest radiograph) remains one of the most commonly ordered imaging study in medicine, yet paradoxically is the most complex. The CXR is difficult to learn, recall, and master effective and accurate interpretation. The chest radiograph is difficult to interpret, especially in critical care where there are usually multiple findings. The chest radiograph includes all thoracic anatomy and provides a high yield, given the low cost and single source.

I would like to point out up front that this work was partially motivated by David S. Feigin, MD, now a professor of radiology at Johns Hopkins University. He is responsible for the systematic analysis of chest radiographs that forms the basis of much of the content of this volume. While a faculty member at the University of California, San Diego (UCSD), he created the Systematic Approach to Pulmonary Abnormalities, which became the scientific content of RoboChest that is used here. He also is responsible for the original Search Pattern for Chest Radiographs, which I have expanded and embellished in this volume, framed in a mnemonic for easy recollection. Dr. Feigin also authored many of the definitions of chest radiology terms that are incorporated herein. Some of the radiographs and other images in this volume are from his collection, including images from the Armed Forces Institute of Pathology, UCSD, the San Diego Veterans Administration Hospital, and USU. I would also like to point out that the work by Squire and Novelline provided the foundation of the systematic diagnostic approach to radiology. [1]

This book is organized by categories of findings that can be seen on the CXR. This material is presented using a directory structure to allow students and residents to dig as deep into details as they like on a topic at hand. In my experience teaching medical students, they seem to recall information more effectively and longer when presented in chunked information segments in a pedagogical fashion. When patterns are repeated, recall is easier from day one; the mindset is prepared for a systematic approach. Otherwise, the CXR remains elusive and often avoided in fear of getting lost in the interpretive process. This book and format should provide a foundation and starting point for fearlessly navigating the CXR consistently from the beginning.

When referring to images or links mentioned in this guide, go to the appropriate webpage using the navigation headings such as the following:

L.R. Folio, *Chest Imaging*, DOI 10.1007/978-1-4614-1317-2_1,
© Henry M. Jackson Foundation for the Advancement of Military Medicine, Inc. 2012

Fundamentals > Chest Primer Presentation

This work presents a structured lexicon for use by students of radiology to repro-ducibly describe abnormalities detected on plain CXRs. The lexicon is designed to provide the students with clinically significant differentiation of abnormalities detected. The content is chunked (displayed) in a directory structure format that relates specific combinations of distinct radiographic findings to classes/groupings of pathological etiologies of those findings. Recognizing the individual findings and identifying their combination or lack of combination with other findings allows one to create effective differential diagnoses that can then be further evaluated using other imaging procedures and/or non-radiographic clinical information. Radiology can be viewed as a descriptive art; where radiologists assign text to the imaging studies. The student of radiology attempts the same process in school, conference, rounds and direct patient care.

Included in this work are hundreds of images including X-rays, Computerized Tomography (CT) images, graphics, analogous models, and animations, to help teach otherwise complex processes and radiographic principles. This material is by no means comprehensive, rather is designed as a teaching tool and entry level infor-mation outlined to select detail and references. This material was not created for medical diagnosis and should not be used in isolation. This book and website can be a launching platform for information on chest imaging.

This directory structure method has been taught in the National Capital Area medi-cal schools and radiology residency programs in the form of categories for years, from the introduction of chest imaging to students, to preparing for boards for senior resi-dents. This method may also be helpful for General Medical Officers (GMOs) in deployed or remote locations without other available references. I have found the intensive care and infectious disease fellows enjoy this organized high-level format and method of solidifying concepts.

Chest X-Ray Interpretation Self-Study Instructions

This Guide organizes the abnormal Chest X-Ray (CXR) into anatomic regions and processes within these regions. This book begins with the search pattern, followed by normal anatomy found on the CXR. A mnemonic-driven approach to the search pattern and diagnostic process allows students, residents, and fellows alike to methodically approach, interpret, and profess the CXR in a quick, efficient, and consistent manner.

Since the CXR has the most anatomic noise (overlapping thoracic skeletal struc-tures, soft tissues, mediastinum, etc.) of any radiographic procedure, the best way I have found to organize this material is to separate out the lungs from everything outside the lungs. Content relating to the lungs can be found in the Abnormal Lung Parenchyma section of the Guide, and content relating to the area outside the lungs is broken up into

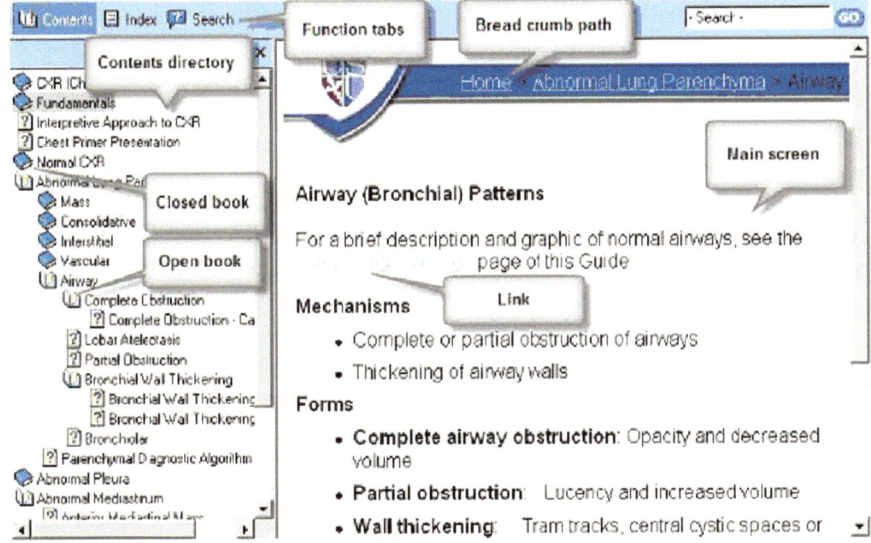

Fig. 1.1 The contents directory is on the left and main screen on the right. At any time, the reader has a breadcrumb trail to show where they are in the algorithm. Image created by USUHS ETI support office

anatomic regions: Abnormal Pleura, Abnormal Mediastinum, and Abnormal Bones, Soft Tissue, and Other Findings. There is also a section about Trauma.

This book and browser tool (available at www.robochest.com) contains search pattern information to determine abnormality and become familiar with abnormal CXRs. Increased familiarity with abnormal CXRs should help guide identification of the general location of the abnormality, which is key to narrowing the differential diagnosis. The tool contains many cases that highlight regional abnormalities. You can match these cases with unknown images in self-study or while on clinical or subspecialty radiology rotations.

Using the RoboChest Website

See Fig. 1.1 for an example screen shot of the RoboChest website. Depending on your browser/security settings, you may need to click a yellow bar at the top of the screen if it appears when you open RoboChest. Clicking this bar and selecting "Allow Blocked Content" will enable your computer to run the ActiveX controls and scripts that are necessary to use RoboChest. The following image shows you an example RoboChest screen described in these instructions.

Once RoboChest is opened, you will note three tabs in the upper left called "Contents," "Index," and "Search." The default tab is "Contents" and will show the directory structure. The Index tab is not yet operational; however, key word searches can be accomplished by using the "Search" tab or the blank text entry on the right top screen.

You will note that the Contents directory works like an interactive table of contents. The book graphics indicate major sections and are "closed" until clicked on, then are "open," with a list of available topic areas or other major headings underneath.

The main screen to the right of the Contents directory structure will display text and graphics aligned with the word or words selected in the Contents directory structure. NOTE: Links open in the main window.

If you click a link (blue, underlined text) on the main screen, the linked content will appear in the main screen, regardless of whether the link takes you to another page in RoboChest or to an outside site. Clicking the back button of your browser will allow you to return to the page that contained the link you clicked.

The main screen will function independently as its own browser window as you dig deeper into the content of your search. No matter what is visible in the main screen, the Contents directory structure will remain on the left and can serve as an outline to keep you focused on the CXR. If you accidentally close it, you can reopen it by clicking the "Contents" tab.

You will note a "bread crumb" path with hyperlinked text within the USU blue banner across the main screen. This path will show your current location in the directory structure while allowing you to click on any higher level for a quick way to see a more broad description of whatever topic you have delved into.

Parenchymal Diagnostic Algorithm (Chest Imaging Diagnostic Algorithm)

The five major lung parenchymal patterns are covered in detail in Chap. 4. Once a student or resident realizes there is a parenchymal process (as opposed to non-parenchymal), then the following patterns help narrow the differential diagnosis. This work was first introduced to the literature in 1993 by Feigin [2].

- *Mass*: Any localized opacity not completely bordered by fissures/pleura
- *Consolidative*: Fluffy, cloud-like, coalescent opacities
- *Interstitial*: Thickening of peribronchial, perivascular, alveolar wall, and/or sub-pleural areas; thick-walled cystic spaces (honeycomb)
- *Vascular*: Change in diameter of vessels, whether intrinsically (vascular volume) or extrinsically (compression such as emphysema)
- *Airway*: Thick-walled airways (circular on end or tram-track), segmental or lobar atelectasis, and, lastly, bronchiectasis

Decision Tree Algorithms to Help Solidify Concepts

Prior work has resulted in two extensive charts in Microsoft® Excel® to help convey the complexity of chest imaging. When one breaks the CXR into components and takes one finding at a time the diagnostic process is simplified.

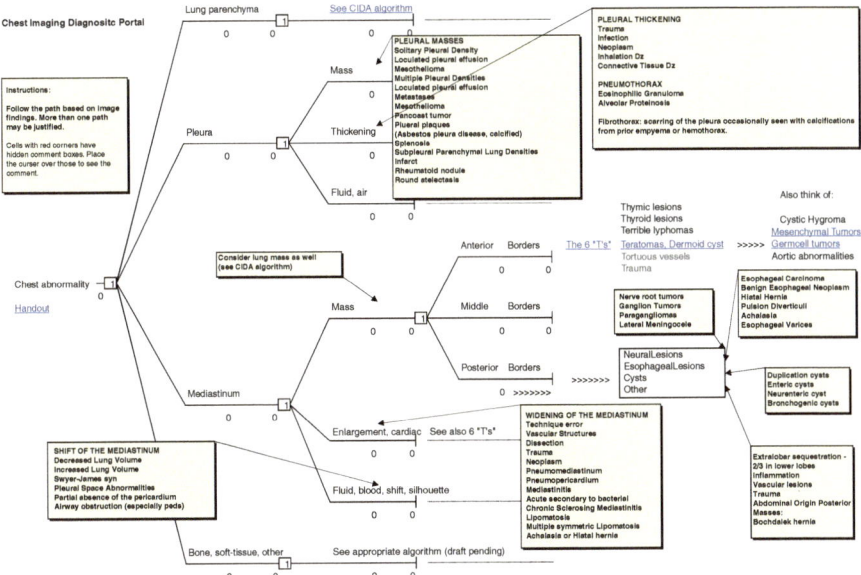

Fig. 1.2 This screen-shot of the higher level algorithm shows all the major anatomic regions where abnormalities can occur in chest imaging. At the top, the "Lung Parenchyma" takes one to the CIDA algorithm (figure 1.3). Both of these algorithms are available on Robochest under "CIDA"

The Chest Imaging Diagnostic Assistant (CIDA) Portal (Fig. 1.2) displays the possible diagnoses for CXR abnormalities. I call this the high level since it leads the other, even more complex algorithm [3]. Abnormalities outside the lungs themselves include the pleural space, mediastinum and components, visualized soft tissues of the chest wall and the included bones. See Fig. 1.3a and b for flowchart for patterns seen in lungs.

You will need to have Microsoft® Excel® installed to view this document in its entirety. You can view this document on www.robochest.com by searching for CIDA. You can then open the document in a new window by clicking the Excel CIDA link and clicking the "Open" button on the download screen. You can also choose to save the document to your computer and view it at a later time.

If you do not have Excel installed but you have a Portable Document Format (PDF) reader such as Adobe® Acrobat®, you can view a PDF version of this document by clicking this PDF CIDA link. Please note, however, that some of the interactive content is not visible in the PDF version.

In summary, this book, along with the RoboChest website, and tools within are intended to enhance the ability of medical students and residents to learn, recall, and

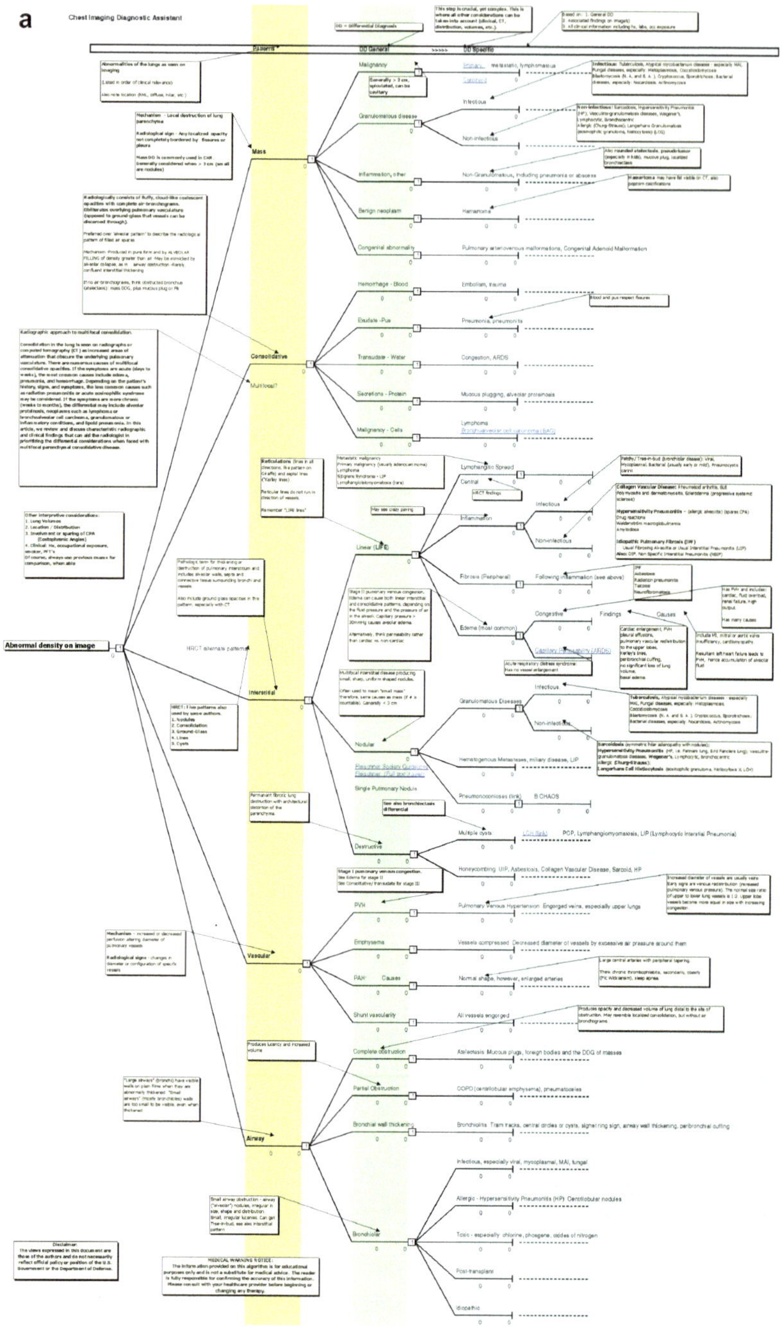

Fig. 1.3 Screen shot (**a**) shows the online Excel® document breaking down the five major lung patterns seen on CXR (Mass, Consolidation, Interstitial, Vascular and Airway patterns). CT and High Resolution CT. Note: this figure is for reference and not meant to be legible. Please refer to the actual document in RoboChest.com under "CIDA"

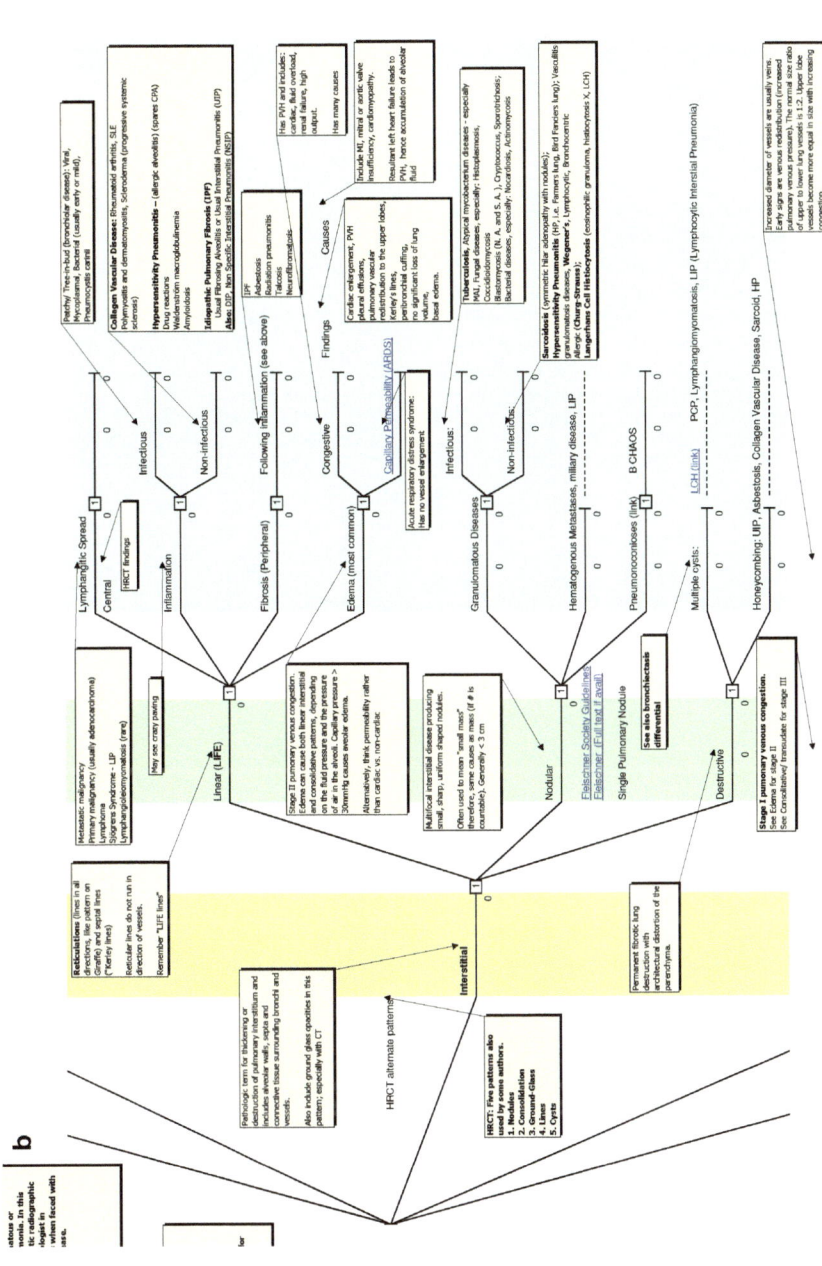

Fig. 1.3 (b) Enlargement of a section of the parenchymal spreadsheet, in this case showing the interstitial pathway magnified section view of the larger chart

master effective Chest X-Ray (CXR) interpretation, and provide a launching platform for chest imaging in general. I hope you enjoy this book and the algorithmic format for learning chest imaging.

References

1. "Squire's Fundamentals of Radiology" 6th edition. Novelline RA. 1964-2004. President and Fellows of Havard College.
2. Feigin DS. A revised system for analysis of abnormal pulmonary images. Chest. 1993;103(2):594–600.
3. Folio L, Feigin DS, Singleton B, Arner D. Algorithmic approach of abnormal patterns in chest imaging: a framework for web-assisted diagnosis. Poster presented at Association of University Radiologists, Knoxville, 2006. p. 82. http://www.aur.org/Annual_Meeting/upload/AUR-2006-Abstracts.pdf. Accessed Sept 2011.

Chapter 2
Search Pattern, Interpretive Approach, Basic Anatomy and Fundamentals

Comprehensive Review of Search Patterns

The following is a concise yet comprehensive review of the Chest X-Ray (CXR) Search Pattern and normal anatomy that should be identified while interpreting the CXR. Based on my teaching experiences and feedback from the first two versions of RoboChest; this chapter is based around the search pattern mnemonic ABCDS×2.

Before starting with the actual search…

- Verify that the patient information and date are complete and accurate on both frontal (PA, Posterior-Anterior, or AP, Anterior-Posterior) and lateral projections (when lateral is available).
- Note position of left or right marker on frontal. Note any inclination markers or secondary indicators of patient positioning. Ask yourself if the patient is upright (do not trust up arrow markers) for example. Be sure you are comparing similar conditions given variable positioning. An effusion one day can look like a consolidation the next, just due to degree of inclination of the patient.
- Note patient position relative to the cassette such as rotation or tilt. The vertebral spinous process should be midway between medial heads of both clavicles. If not, take this into consideration as relative densities may change.
- Note adequacy of penetration or other potential technical defects. For example, you should be able to see intervertebral disk space through the heart shadow.
- Look briefly at the entirety of both projections for obvious abnormalities.

L.R. Folio, *Chest Imaging*, DOI 10.1007/978-1-4614-1317-2_2,
© Henry M. Jackson Foundation for the Advancement of Military Medicine, Inc. 2012

Search Pattern Mnemonic

The CXR search pattern should be systematic and the approach to the CXR should be methodic [1], applying the normal anatomy, principles, information, and examples mentioned in the "Normal Anatomy."

The student of radiology should have a mental checklist that is easily recalled each time a CXR is reviewed. It is important to get into a routine and check everything on the images.

The mnemonic [2] in Table 2.1 is like the popular ABCs in life support, only two at a time AA, BB, CC, DD, SS.

Table 2.1 (ABCDs)2

A – Airway	A – Aorta
B – Breathing	B – Bones
C – Circulation	C – Cardiac
D – Diaphragm	D – Deformity
S – Soft tissues	S – Shoulder

This simple mnemonic can be applied to reviewing the CXR. One mentally goes through this checklist as a pilot approaches a landing in a methodical, mandated challenge and response. For example, following assurance that the correct patient is being evaluated and technical factors are considered, one says "Airway" quietly to themselves and looks at the airway for abnormalities, then says "Aorta" then follows the aortic shadow (based on information provided in the normal anatomy section that follows), and so on. When a lateral is available, the mnemonic is repeated; hence this duplicated "ABCDs" is repeated

Interpretive Approach to CXR

Once an abnormality (often more than one) is detected using either search pattern described in this section of this Guide, a systematic process should be applied to come to a working differential diagnosis.

The following mnemonic may help approach interpretation of chest radiographs and clinical image reasoning in a methodical fashion: *ID CD* Table 2.2.

Table 2.2 The diagnostic approach to each chest x-ray, or CT for that matter, should be methodical and standard. Following the IDCD format should provide a framework to arrive at a differential diagnosis with all findings, hence categories in mind

ID CD of systematic approach to radiographic interpretation:
I – Identify the abnormality and localize anatomically.
D – Define the appearance (be descriptive: margins, density, etc.).
C – Categorize or classify into patterns, grades.
D – Differential diagnosis.

You will notice most cases in this book will follow a similar format to the above ID CD. Sticking to this (or a similar) process may help in class, conferences, board exams, and eventually and most importantly, with the patient under consideration.

Fig. 2.1 The normal chest X-ray, PA (posterior to anterior) view

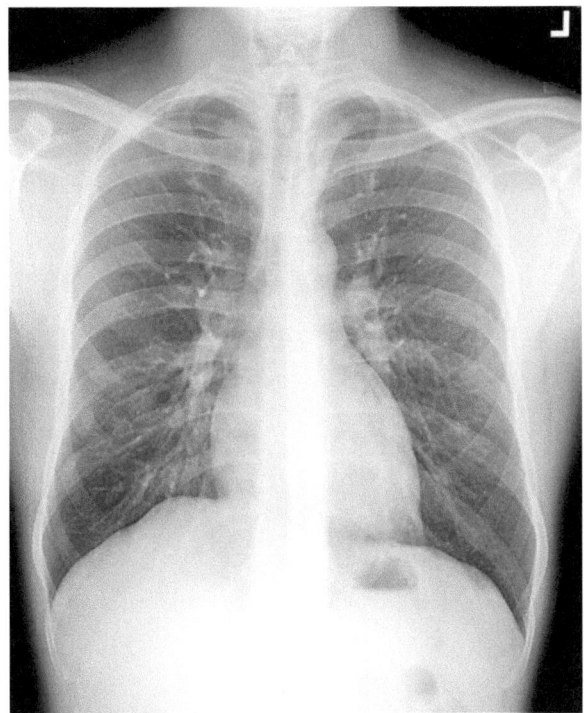

Applying the Mnemonic to the Search Pattern

Details to consider on each of the items:
  Frontal view (also known as either the PA posterior-anterior, or AP)

- *Airway*: Follow the trachea to the carina and main bronchi.
- *Aorta*: Follow the aortic contour.
- *Breathing*: Study the lungs, both up and down and side to side. Include lung volumes and symmetry of markings. Check the periphery of the lungs for pneumothorax and effusions.
- *Bones*: Assess all ribs and visible spine.
- *Circulation*: Look at both hila (pulmonary arteries for the most part) for enlargement and abnormal bulges.
- *Cardiac*: Evaluate mediastinal contours, edges, and shape.
- *Diaphragm*: Check both hemidiaphragms for blunting, shape, and position. Also check upper abdomen for free air and abnormal air collections.
- *Deformity*: Again assess spine for any deformity such as scoliosis, pedicle asymmetry.
- *Soft tissues*: Trace the periphery of the chest, outside the lungs and ribs (chest wall). Include visible portions of soft tissues of the neck.
- *Shoulder*: Look at the shoulders specifically, soft tissue and bones, especially on the frontal projection.

Fig. 2.2 The normal chest
X-ray, lateral view

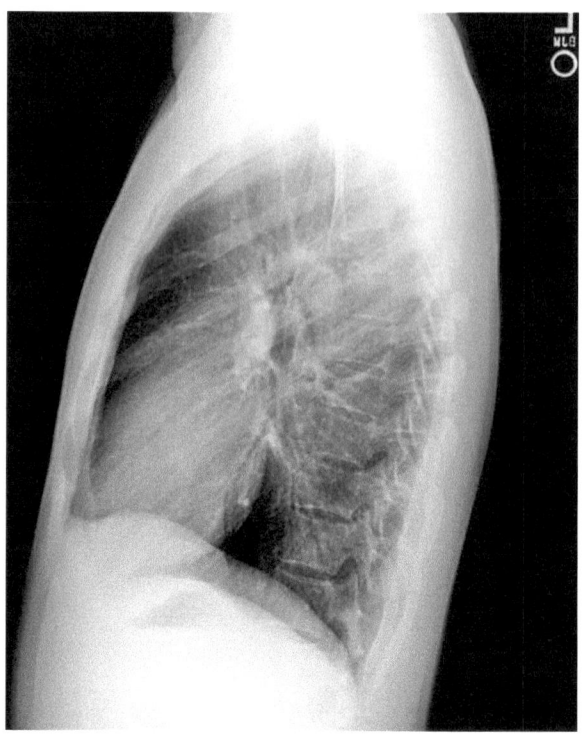

Lateral view

- *Airway*: Follow the trachea to the left main bronchus.
- *Aorta*: Follow the aortic contour.
- *Breathing*: Review lung volumes and overall appearance. Check the periphery (anterior and posterior) of the lungs for pneumothorax and effusions/ loculations.
- *Bones*: Follow the spine downward for vertebral bodies and darkening. Also assess all ribs.
- *Circulation*: Note the size and shape of pulmonary arteries.
- *Cardiac*: Note the area posterior to the heart and the darkening one should see toward the diaphragm. Evaluate mediastinal contours, edges, and shape. Look upward for darkening of the anterior mediastinum to the neck.
- *Diaphragm*: Judge the size and shape of the diaphragms. Check the upper abdomen for free air and abnormal air collections.
- *Deformity*: Assess spine for any deformity such as increased or decreased kyphosis, wedge shapes (compression or pathological fractures).
- *Soft tissues*: Trace the periphery of the chest, outside the lungs and ribs (chest wall). Include visible portions of soft tissues of the neck and abdomen.
- *Shoulder*: Consider the boney and soft tissue shoulder effects on the lateral.

Note that on the lateral, there are three areas of progressive lucency. This is described in detail recently by Feigin [3].

1. As you scan from the back of heart to the costophrenic angles, there should be progressive darkening.
2. As you scan from the anterior mediastinum to the sternum (retrosternal clear space)
3. As you scan along down spine along vertebral bodies, it should get darker.

Deviation from the above progressive lucencies may indicate pathology and should trigger attention.

Chest Primer Presentation

The Chest Primer Presentation is a self-paced guide to CXR interpretation. It can be viewed on RoboChest (search for "Primer"). If you have Microsoft® PowerPoint® or PowerPoint Viewer installed, you can use the interactive version by clicking this PowerPoint Chest Primer Presentation link, clicking the "Open" button on the download screen, and then choosing the "Slide Show" view in PowerPoint to view the slides. The presentation will open in a new window. You can also choose to save the presentation to your computer and view the slide show at a later time. If you do not have PowerPoint installed but you have a Portable Document Format (PDF) reader such as Adobe® Acrobat®, you can view this presentation as a PDF by clicking this PDF Chest Primer Presentation link.

References

1. Halvorsen JG, Swanson D. Interpreting office radiographs. A guide to systematic evaluation. J Fam Pract. 1990;31(6):602–10.
2. Folio LR. A mnemonic approach to the evaluation of chest X-ray films. J Am Osteopath Assoc. 1995;95(11):648.
3. Feigin DS. Lateral chest radiograph a systematic approach. Acad Radiol. 2010;17(12):1560–6.

Chapter 3
Normal Chest X-Ray, Terminology and Radiographic Anatomy

Introduction and Terminology

The chest X-Ray (CXR) usually consists of two views: the PA (Posterior to Anterior) and the lateral. Figures 3.1 and 3.2 are example PA and lateral views without pathology. Other figures in this chapter will show you the different elements of the normal anatomy as they appear in a normal CXR.

The CXR includes everything in the thorax and has a high yield given the low cost and single source. This section of the book highlights the normal anatomy seen on CXRs.

Chest Imaging Terminology

Here are some important terms related to the CXR.

Conspicuity: Degree of "conspicuous-ness" or visibility.
High conspicuity is an obvious finding, and a decreased conspicuity is a subtle finding. Various properties or adjacent structures may alter conspicuity.

Consolidation: Air space opacities that are fluffy (like cumulous clouds) that often indicate pneumonia. This is described in more detail in the lung parenchyma chapter.

Density: Whiteness, or any area of whiteness, on an image (opacity). Bones are an example. Imaging densities also include soft tissues including, blood/fluid, fat, calcium and even air low density.

Edge: Any visible demarcation between a density on one side and lucency on the other.
An important X-Ray phenomenon is that the edge of a structure is only visible if it is bordered by a structure of different density.

L.R. Folio, *Chest Imaging*, DOI 10.1007/978-1-4614-1317-2_3,

Fig. 3.1 Normal PA
(or frontal) chest radiograph

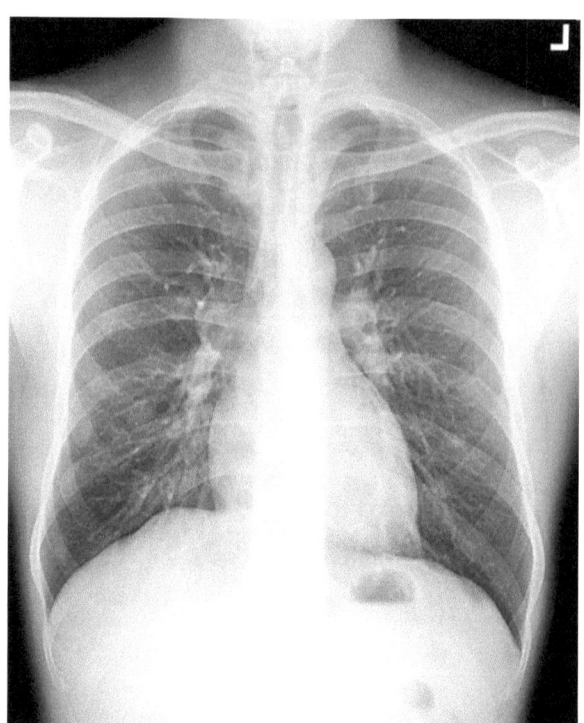

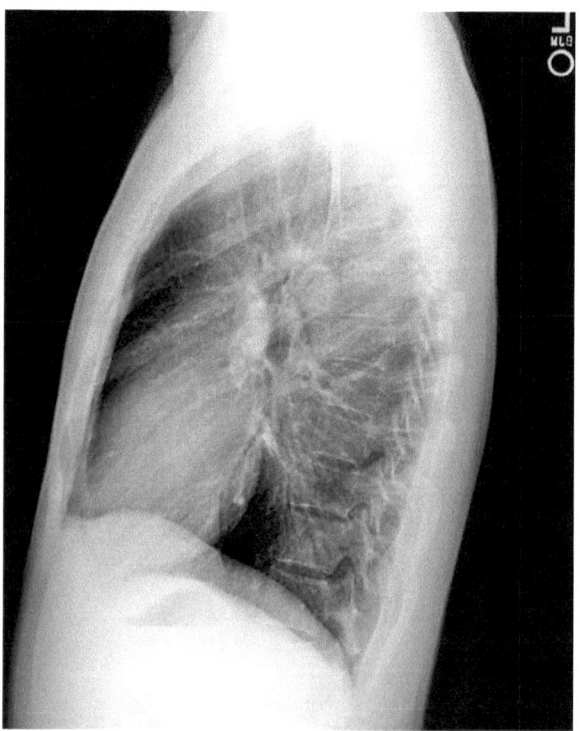

Fig. 3.2 Normal left lateral
chest radiograph

Fig. 3.3 Radiograph of syringe showing line versus an edge. Also note the fluid/fluid level (*water/contrast*) of this syringe taken in the upright position with the X-Ray tube (*hence the beam*) horizontal relative to gravity

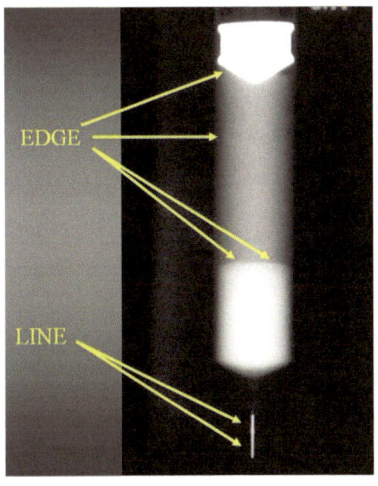

En Face: Indicates orientation of structure; think of a swallowed coin in the esophagus. The "face" would be seen on the frontal projection (due to esophagus orientation) and the edge would be seen on the lateral (profile or on-end).

Fluid level: An edge between a dependent fluid and adjacent air (air-fluid level) or another fluid of differing density (fluid-fluid level). Only seen on erect projections with horizontal beam. See Fig. 3.3.

Horizontal beam: When the X-Ray tube is horizontally oriented relative to the patient and the X-Ray beam is parallel to the floor. This is the only way to effectively demonstrate a fluid level.

Infiltrate: A non-descript term that is often used to indicate an opacity exists that may represent a consolidation, interstitial pattern or atelectasis. From the radiologist to the provider, there is flexibility in interpretation.

Interstitial: Used to describe linear opacities that are not vessels; rather may cross vessels at angles not in branching patterns. This is described in more detail in the lung parenchyma chapter.

Line: A thin density with lucency on both sides or a thin lucency with density on both sides.

Lucency: Blackness, or any area of blackness, on an image. The trachea is an example.

Mach (not mock) bands (or effect): Center-surround receptive field interactions resulting in apparent lucencies. These often occur adjacent to curved densities next to relative lucencies (such as the right atrial heart shadow).

Mass: A well defined opacity that may or may not represent a mass (e.g., tumor verses a pseudotumor).

Obliterated: Obscured structure that should otherwise be seen. Other descriptions include "masked," "not seen" or "not well discerned".

Projection: the path of the X-Ray beam, can be a frontal projection (either PA or AP), lateral, decube, or upright (erect) etc.

Shadow: Anything visible on an image; hence, any specific density or lucency.

Silhouette: Synonym for edge. Loss of an edge constitutes the "silhouette sign." This occurs by adjacent structures masking others; such as how a right middle lobe (RML) consolidation obliterates the right atrial edge.

Stripe: Either an edge or a line.

Summation Shadow: Anatomic noise of overlapping structures. This often happens with posterior ribs overlapping vessels and anterior ribs; mimicking an infiltrate.

Tram tracks: Parallel lines that look like tram (or train) tracks due to their outlining bronchi in bronchiectasis.

There are many important elements in the description of a finding. They include the following.

- Anatomic location: such as distribution, lobar, diffuse, central
- Proximity: for example adjacent to, surrounded by (think 2D image of 3D anatomy).
- Pattern: examples include mass, consolidate, etc.
- Orientation: such as en-face (face-on), profile (opposite of en-face)
- Angle of approximation: obtuse vs. acute angle

See Fig. 3.3 that demonstrates a fluid-fluid level along with a few other terms described. This is a radiograph of a syringe oriented vertically with immiscible contrast (more dense and dependent) and water (less dense on top) showing an edge at the interface. Note that the needle represents a line (which is thinner than an edge).

Mach Effect on CXR

The following series of images shows the Mach effect, a very common phenomenon seen on chest X-Rays [1].

In Fig. 3.4, the apparent lucency next to the edge (of skin) in the right lung field is actually a Mach band. The skin fold is not uncommon in portable CXRs in that the plate is sometimes moved up to get the apicies, pulling exposed skin up. This creates an edge with associated lucency (Fig. 3.5), which actually represents the Mach effect. Figures 3.6 and 3.7 show close-ups of the Mach effect.

Trachea and Lungs on CXR

Figures 3.8–3.11 highlight the appearance of the trachea and lungs on a normal CXR.

Fig. 3.4 This demonstrates how the Mach effect can mimic a pneumothorax

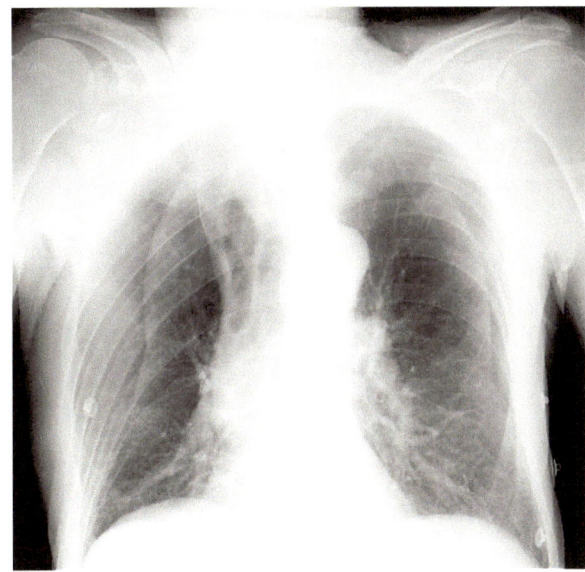

Fig. 3.5 See close up of skin fold with apparent lucency adjacent to the fold edge

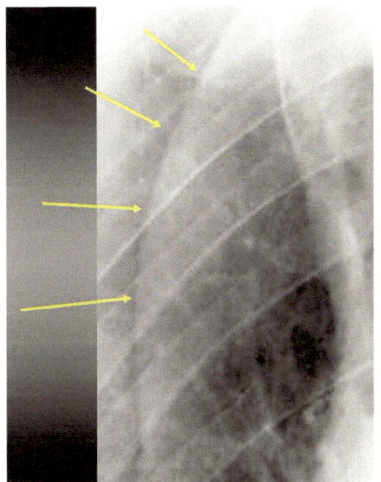

Mediastinal Anatomy on CXR

The heart and great vessels make up a majority of the mediastinal silhouette on the frontal CXR. Figures 3.12–3.16 highlight the elements of mediastinal anatomy on the CXR.

The aortic knob on the left is formed by the superior and outer edge of the aortic arch.

The cardiac silhouette on normal chest X-Rays is made up of the right atrium on the right and the left ventricle on the left. The posterior edge seen on the lateral is due to the left ventricle.

Fig. 3.6 Mach band bordering right atrium

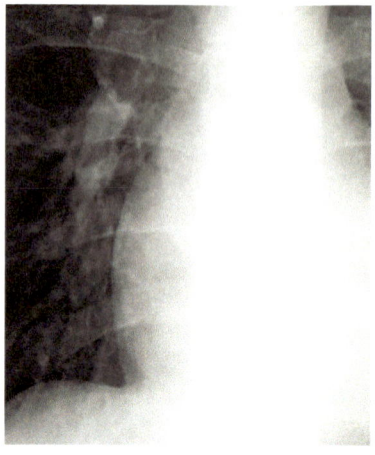

Fig. 3.7 Mach band bordering right atrium, indicated by *arrows*

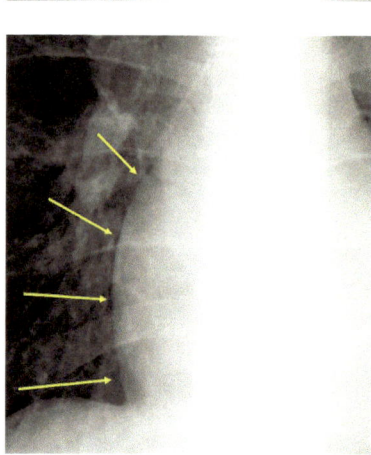

The Hilum (Plural: Hila)

The hila are the anatomic connections of the lung to the mediastinum and consist of a variety of vessels, bronchi, and lymph nodes.

In Figs. 3.17 and 3.18, the visible portion of each normal hilum is the right or left pulmonary artery. The pulmonary veins are inferior and posterior to the arteries, behind the edges of the heart on the frontal view and overlapping many other structures on the lateral view. The major bronchi are visible as lucencies. The lymph nodes are too small to be visible, at least when they are normal. When there is hilar bulky adenopathy, however, this can be seen as lumpy, enlarged hila.

The right and left pulmonary arteries are visible on the lateral view, in the center of the image. The right pulmonary artery is just anterior to the air column (trachea continuous with main bronchi) and the left pulmonary artery is just posterior.

See Fig. 3.19 for where to look for the Main Pulmonary Artery (MPA) on the PA projection; when present.

Fig. 3.8 The trachea that is visible on chest X-Ray is outlined with *red lines*

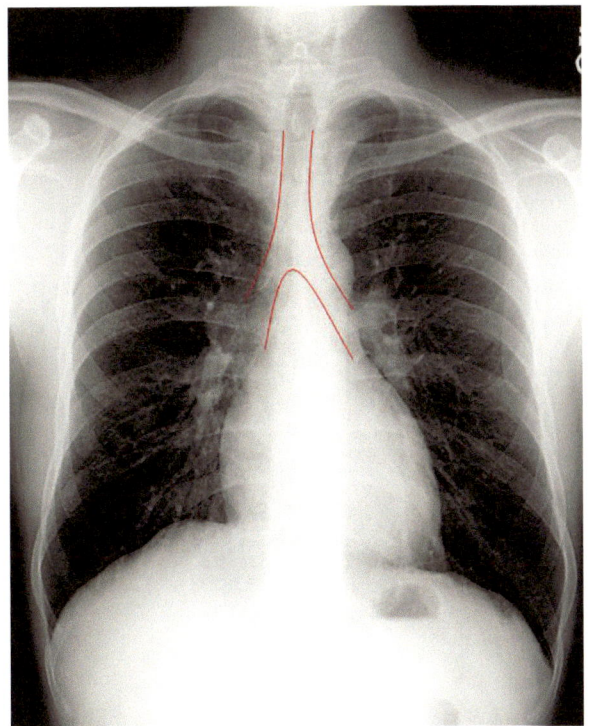

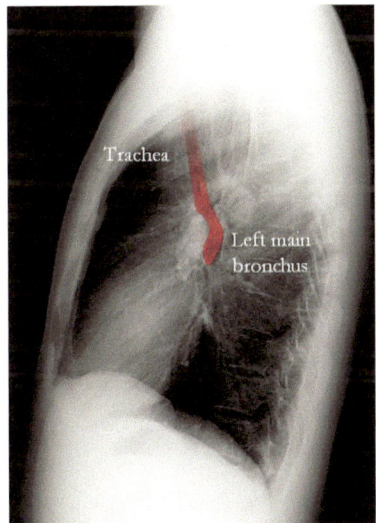

Fig. 3.9 Trachea that should be visible on the lateral projection is seen in *red*. The visible trachea on the lateral terminates at the left main bronchus (seen as a *lucent circle*). Key: *RUL* right upper lobe, *RML* right middle lobe, *RLL* right lower lobe, *LUL* left upper lobe, *LLL* left lower lobe

Fig. 3.10 Lung lobes colored to show overlap on the PA. Note, the diaphragm borders the lower lobes giving the curvilinear appearance. Key: *RUL* right upper lobe, *RML* right middle lobe, *RLL* right lower lobe, *LUL* left upper lobe, *LLL* left lower lobe

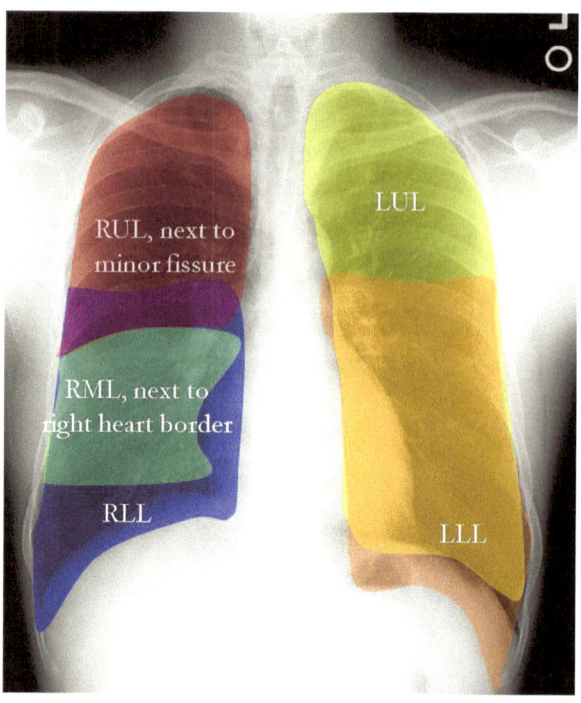

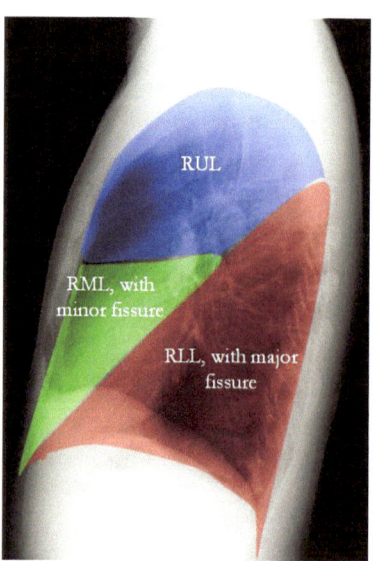

Fig. 3.11 The right lung lobes on lateral. The left would be just left upper lobe (no right middle lobe, but including that region)

Fig. 3.12 Superior vena cava (SVC) edge and left paratracheal stripe

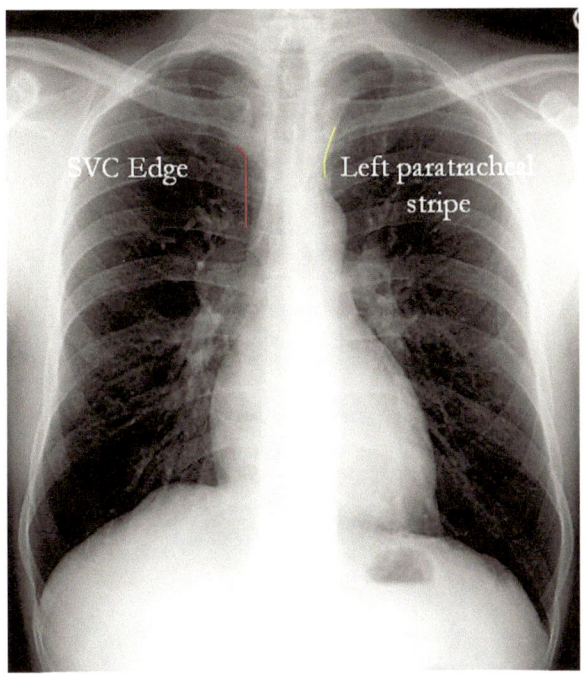

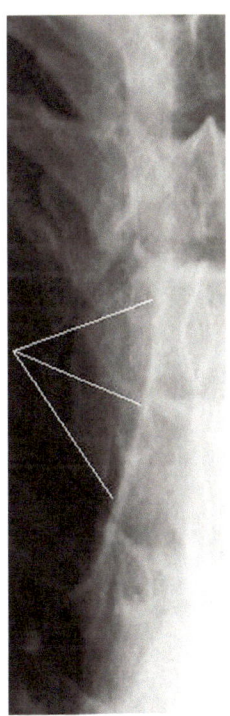

Fig. 3.13 Close-up of the paratracheal line. Note: this is not always appreciated on portables

Fig. 3.14 Aorta as seen on PA projection is filled in *red*

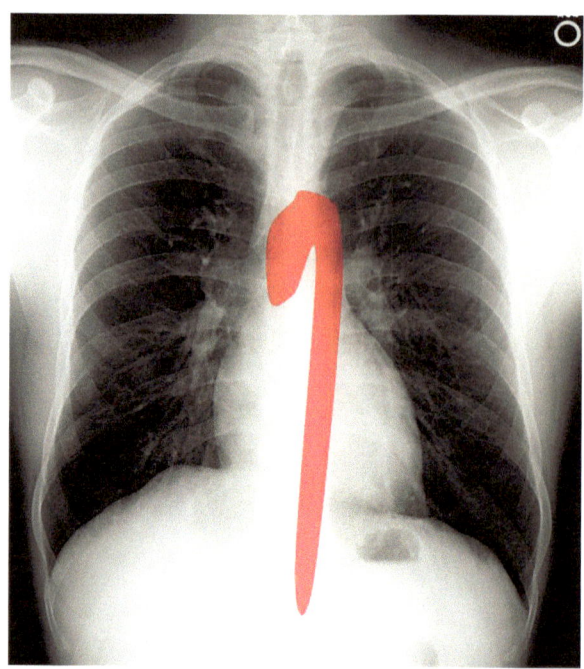

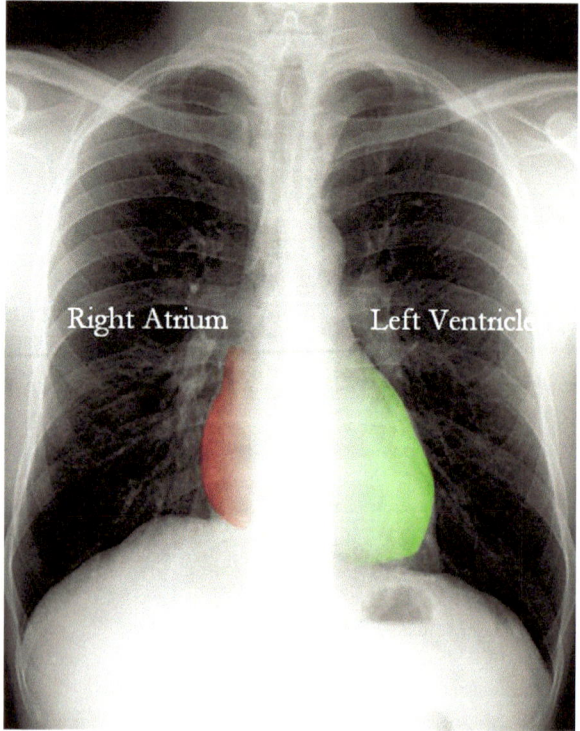

Fig. 3.15 Right atrium (*red*) and left ventricle (*green*) on the PA

Fig. 3.16 Right atrium (*red*) and left ventricle (*green*) on the lateral

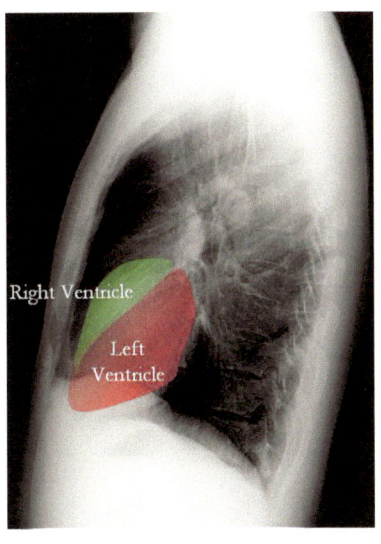

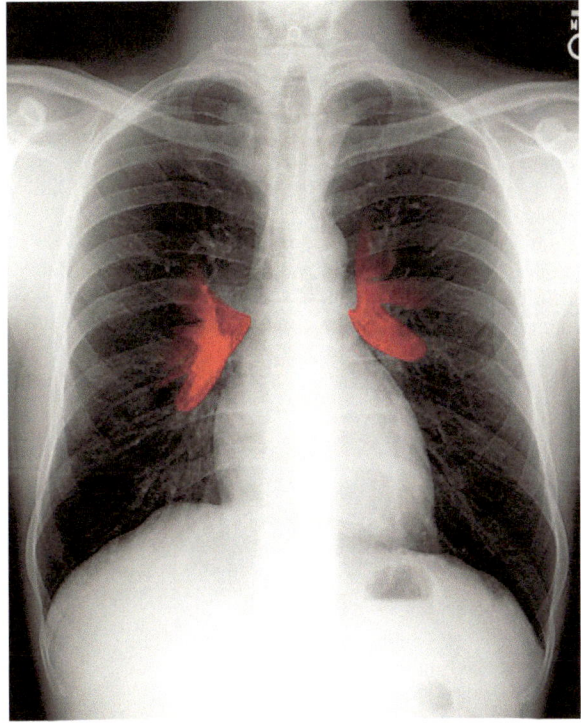

Fig. 3.17 The normal Hila shown here in *red*

Fig. 3.18 Hila (*again in red*), along with aorta (*yellow*) on lateral

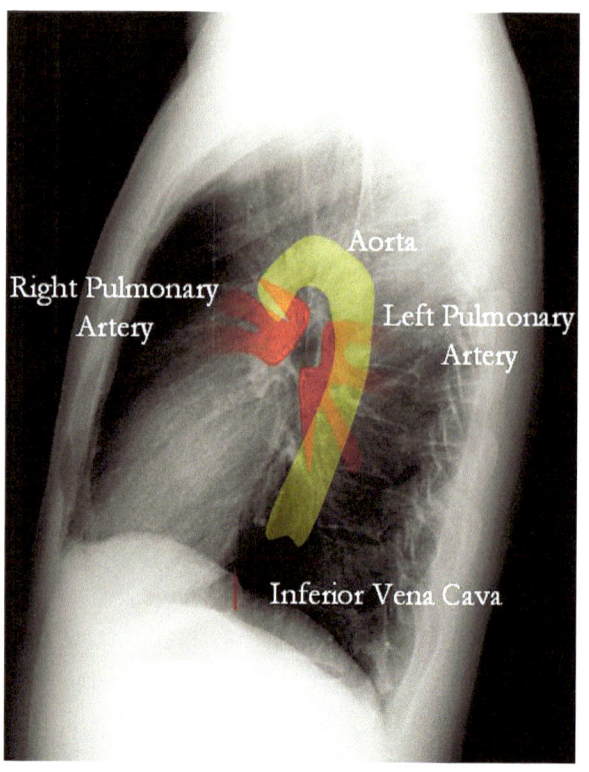

Fig. 3.19 Main pulmonary artery (MPA) outlined with the short *yellow curved line*

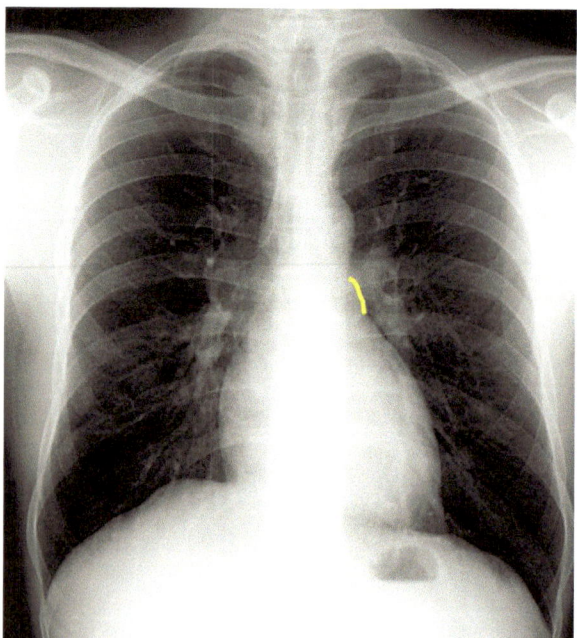

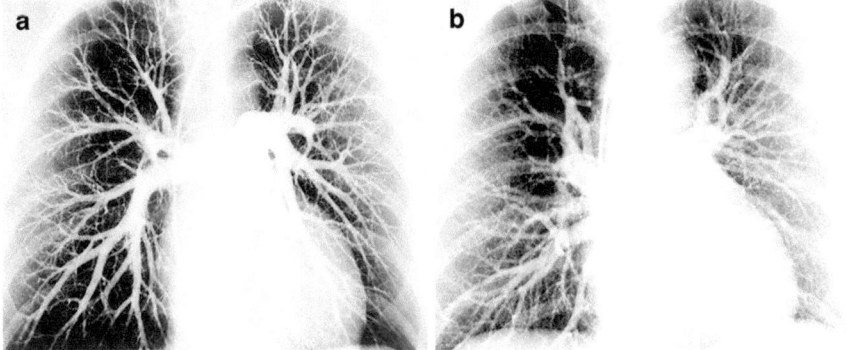

Fig. 3.20 (**a**) Pulmonary angiogram in the arterial phase; (**b**) Pulmonary angiogram in the venous phase; showing the more inferior location of the pulmon ary veins

Pulmonary Arteries and Veins

See (Figs. 3.20 a-d) for pulmonary angiogram images, obtained after the administration of a contrast injection into the pulmonary arteries directly (note the catheter). Note how the main pulmonary arteries (left image) are more superior than the major veins (right image, taken about 20 s after first image). The confluence of the pulmonary veins are inferior and posterior to origin of the pulmonary arteries. See Fig. 3.21 showing approximate location of pulmonary veins on PA view.

Normal Lung Markings

The only normal densities within the lungs are the pulmonary vessels when filled with blood and fissures. Where they are seen, they are densities, not lucencies.

Vessel Size

Vessels in the lungs may appear as small nodules. The following helps differentiate normal vessels from nodules.

Vessels on-end should be the same size as similarly distributed vessels in profile: i.e., expected size/compared size. In the following image, note that the vessel on-end (circled) is about the same size as the vessel seen leading to it (between lines, below the circled vessel).

Normal pulmonary markings (vessels) can be followed from the hilum toward the lung periphery in all directions. They branch at acute angles, taper and diverge toward the periphery.

Abnormal pulmonary markings are any shadows in the area of lungs that are IN ADDITION to the normal markings (fissures, vessels).

Many such shadows obscure the normal markings or displace them.

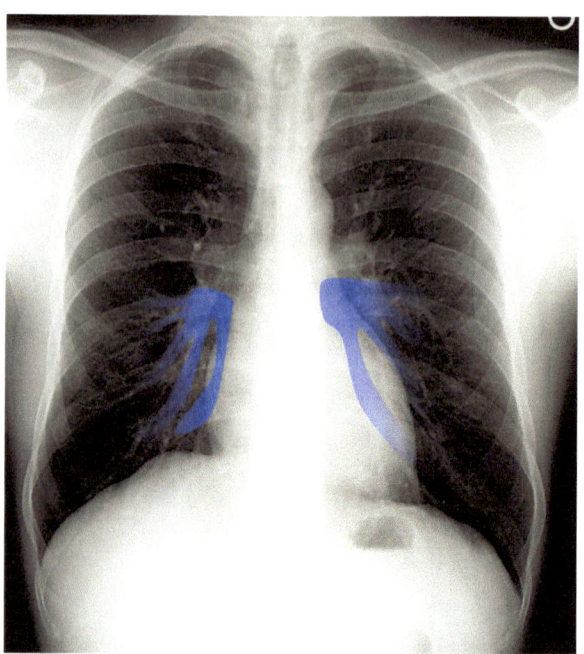

Fig. 3.21 Pulmonary veins colored *blue* here. Note these are inferior to the pulmonary arteries

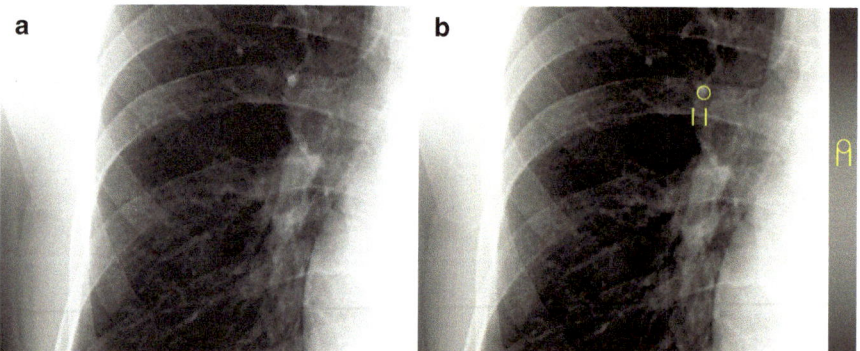

Fig. 3.22 Comparing vessel size on end to differentiate from nodules. The expected vessel size on end (*circle*) should be the same as the visible vessel (*two lines*). When larger, the density may represent a nodule. Figure **b** has the annotations for figure **a**

Fig. 3.23 Azygoesophageal
edge

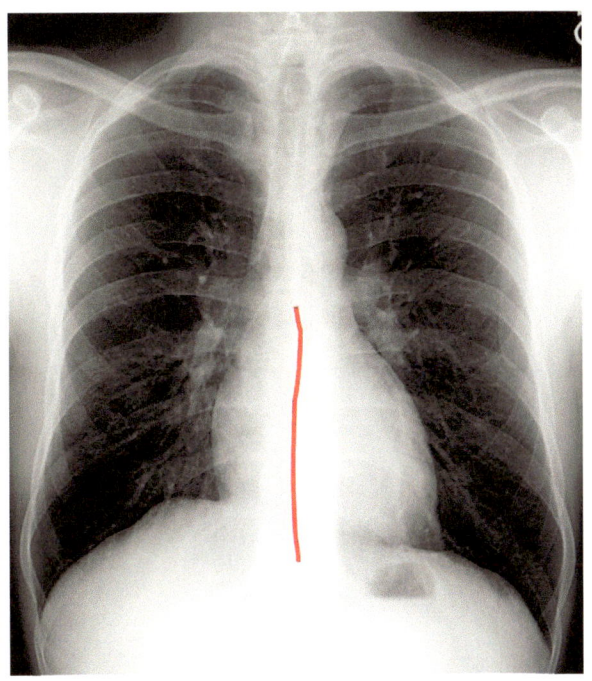

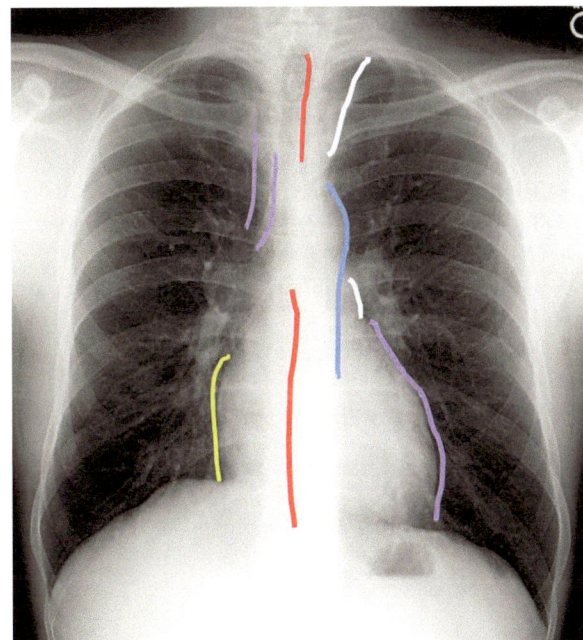

Fig. 3.24 PA chest with *lines*
outlining mediastinal
structures. Match with the list
of structures before looking
at answers on following page

Fig. 3.25 PA chest with *lines* numbered according to anatomy listed *above*

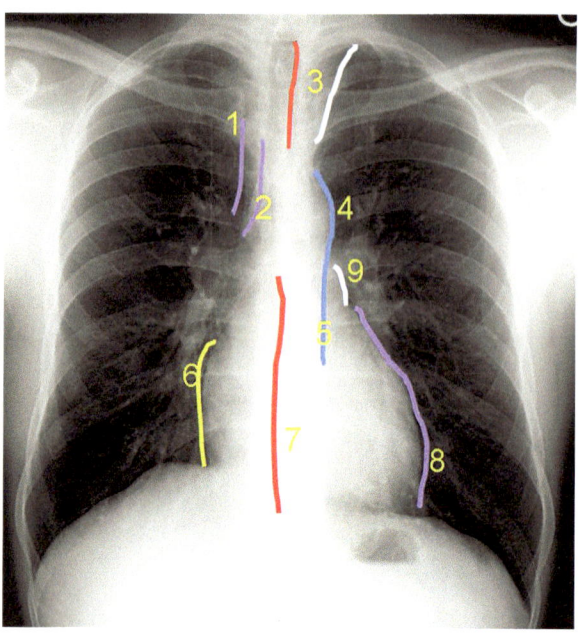

Quiz Yourself: Mediastinum Lines, Edges

Using the number assigned to each item, match the items on Fig. 3.25 in the list below to the lines in the image. It is recommended that you test yourself before advancing to the answers.

Mediastinal structures on the PA CXR

1. SVC Edge
2. Right Paratracheal Line
3. Left Paratracheal Stripe (both red and white lines)
4. Aortic Arch
5. Descending Aorta (only left edge seen, and not always)
6. Right Atrium
7. Azygoesophageal edge
8. Left Ventricle
9. Main Pulmonary Artery (also known as: trunk, middle mogul)

Fig. 3.26 Close-up of
shoulder on frontal projection
showing skeletal anatomy
that can be identified

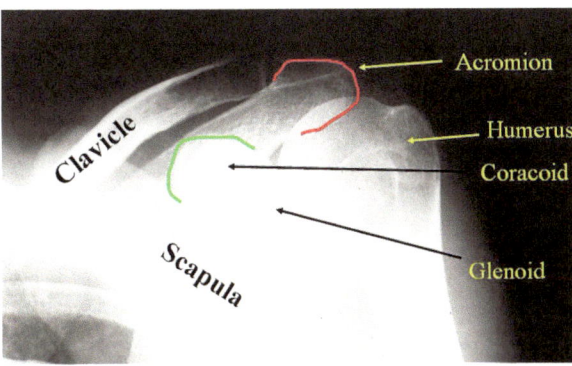

Shoulder Anatomy

Figure 3.26 highlights the anatomy of the shoulder often seen on a normal CXR.

Reference

1. Hall FM. Mach band theory. Radiology. 2001;221(3):850.

Chapter 4
Abnormal Lung Patterns

Abnormal Lung Parenchyma

As mentioned in the normal CXR section, the only structures visible in normal lungs are the fissures and pulmonary vessels. Any other structures visible are likely abnormalities. This section breaks down lung parenchymal abnormalities into five basic patterns that have been previously described, and taught in the National Capital Area residencies for years [1]:

1. Mass
2. Consolidative
3. Interstitial
4. Vascular
5. Airway

It should be kept in mind this is a findings-based approach and not the actual pathology that underlies the finding. For example, a mass finding is not always a "mass" in that abnormal vessels (e.g., AVM, rounded atelectasis or pneumonia, or aberrant vessels) may resemble a mass that represents vasculature or other process. Similarly, the vascular pattern may be primarily an abnormality of lung tissue surrounding the vessels causing compression or distortion, hence a secondary vascular effect. In other words, vessel distortion/alteration may be the only clue to the abnormality.

Mass

An opacity is classified as a mass when it is reasonably well defined and is not the shape of any anatomic structure of the lung, such as a complete lobe or segment. An opacity is also a mass when its borders are not entirely composed of fissures or the

L.R. Folio, *Chest Imaging*, DOI 10.1007/978-1-4614-1317-2_4,
© Henry M. Jackson Foundation for the Advancement of Military Medicine, Inc. 2012

Fig. 4.1 Example of a parenchymal mass. This well marinated, rounded opacity also displays the hilar overlay sign in that the hilar vessels can be seen through the mass

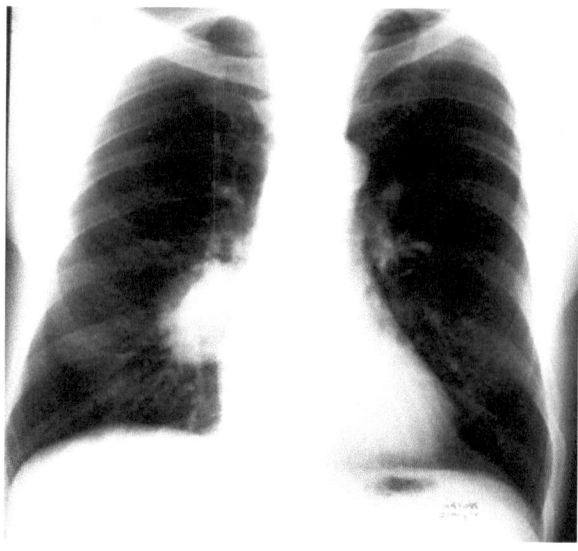

pleura; that may make the process resemble a mass (well-defined border, for example). Masses are usually rounded or ovoid.

See Fig. 4.1 for an example CXR with a mass in the right hilum. This ended up being a carcinoid.

Mass Considerations

Two considerations to think about when identifying a mass are the size of the mass as compared to normal vasculature and the shape of the mass.

Size

As previously mentioned, vessels in the lungs may appear as small nodules. These are important to differentiate from vessels. Vessels on-end should be the same size as similarly distributed vessels in profile: i.e., expected size/compared size.

Mass Characteristics

There are a few clues to narrowing down the mass differential. These include size, shape, margins, number, and distribution [2]. Many masses seen on CXR end up being evaluated CT [3].

Fig. 4.2 Benign calcification patterns (Image created by USUHS ETI Support Office)

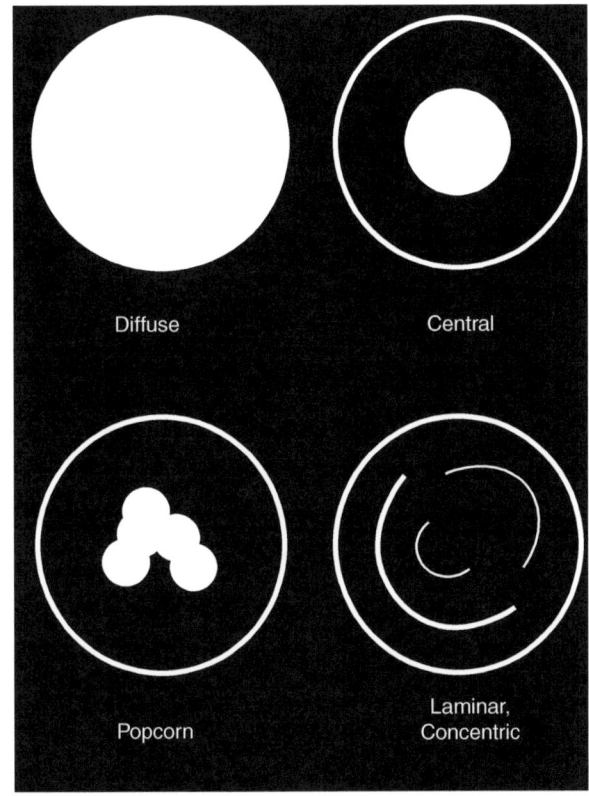

Fig. 4.3 Indeterminate (potentially malignant) calcification patterns (Image created by USUHS ETI Support Office)

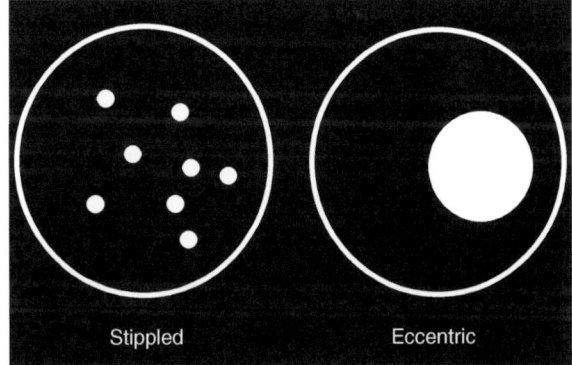

Calcification Distribution in Masses

Calcifications are commonly visible in CXRs of Solitary Pulmonary Nodules (SPNs).

Fig. 4.4 Primary lung
carcinoma

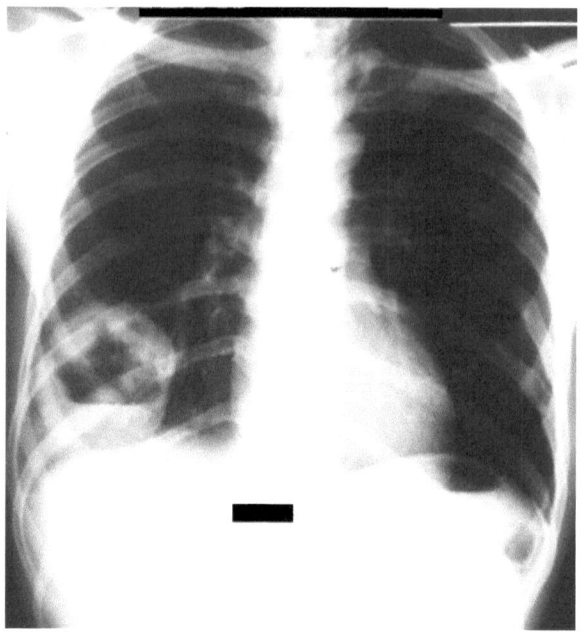

"Organized patterns of calcification, such as 'popcorn' (seen in hamartomas), lamellar concentric rings of calcium, central calcification, or homogeneous dense calcification, all carry an extremely low likelihood of malignancy [4]."

"Not all nodules that contain calcification are benign. Certain patterns of calcification are considered radiologically 'indeterminate,' meaning that they do not increase or decrease the likelihood of malignancy compared to a non-calcified nodule. These indeterminate patterns include stippled fine calcification and eccentric calcification."

Malignancy

There are two general categories of lung cancer: Large cell carcinomas (which are usually classified as non-small cell types) and small cell carcinoma. Non-small cell lung cancer (NSCLC) accounts for approximately 75% of all lung cancers. Of note, bronchoalveolar cell carcinoma (BAC) and lymphoma can display as a consolidative pseudo-mass.

Case 4.1

Figures 4.4 and 4.5 show an example of a primary lung carcinoma.

Fig. 4.5 Primary lung carcinoma, lateral view

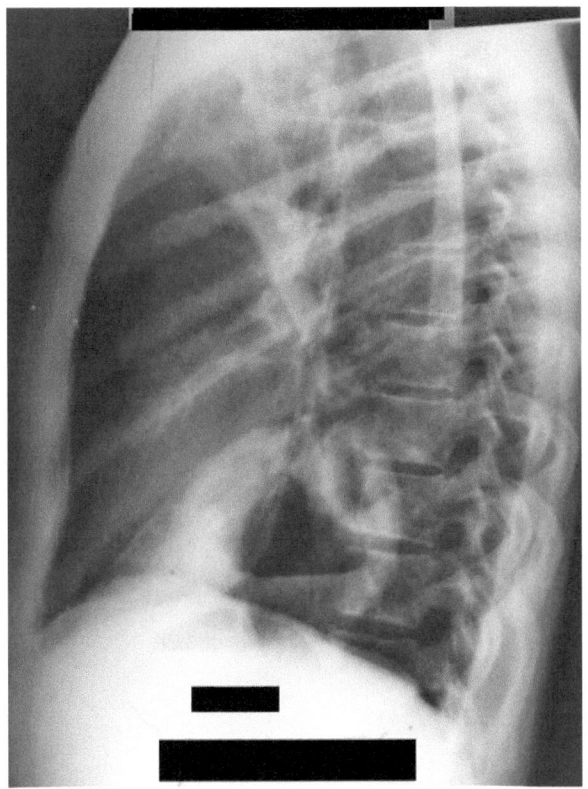

Findings: A cavitated round opacity is present at the right lung base. It overlies the back of the heart shadow on the lateral view. The location is thus right lower lobe. There are nodular opacities inside the cavity and an air-fluid level is visible.

Pattern: This is a mass pattern.

Differential Diagnosis: Malignancy is favored over inflammation because of the irregularity of the inner wall of the cavity. The air-fluid level is not useful in differential diagnosis; it only indicates that the bronchus connected to the mass is either partially or intermittently obstructed.

Diagnosis: Bronchogenic carcinoma, adenomatous.

Metastatic

Characteristics like shape, distribution, and multiplicity support metastatic mass diagnosis. Normal pulmonary markings (vessels) can be followed from the hilum toward the lung periphery in all directions. They branch at acute angles, taper, and diverge toward the periphery.

Fig. 4.6 PA showing multiple nodules on left (all less than 3 cm) and nodules and one mass on the right (3.4 cm)

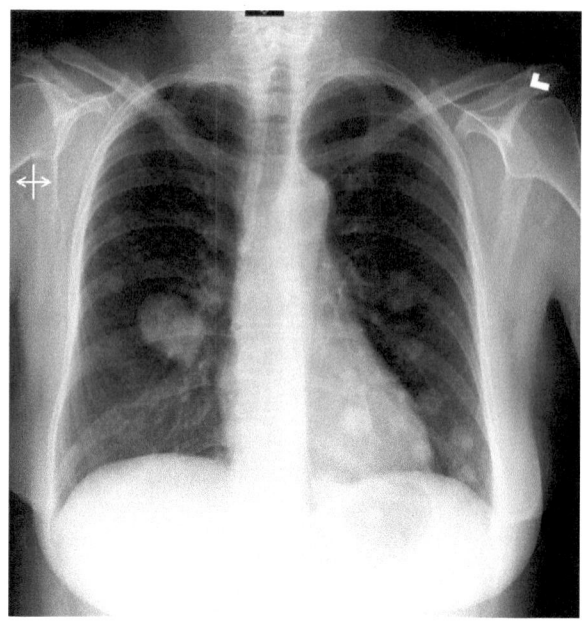

Case 4.2

This case (Figs. 4.6 – 4.8) depicts multiple metastatic masses.
   Findings: Multiple well-rounded opacities in the left lung.
   Pattern: Mass (and nodules), multiple, bilateral.

Differential Diagnosis
- Malignancy
- Granulomatous disease
- Inflammation
- Benign neoplasm
- Congenital

   Since there are multiple masses, malignancy (metastatic), granulomatous, and congenital become higher on the differential. Given a history of adrenal cortical carcinoma, metastatic is the primary diagnosis. Metastatic is the highest on the differential.

Bronchial Carcinoid

Bronchial Carcinoid lesions are classified from low grade (typical) to high grade (atypical). Both extremes have similar imaging features, with the majority of lesions being centrally located, well-defined, and round-to-ovoid in shape.

Fig. 4.7 Lateral demonstrating the mass overlying the hilum and multiple nodules

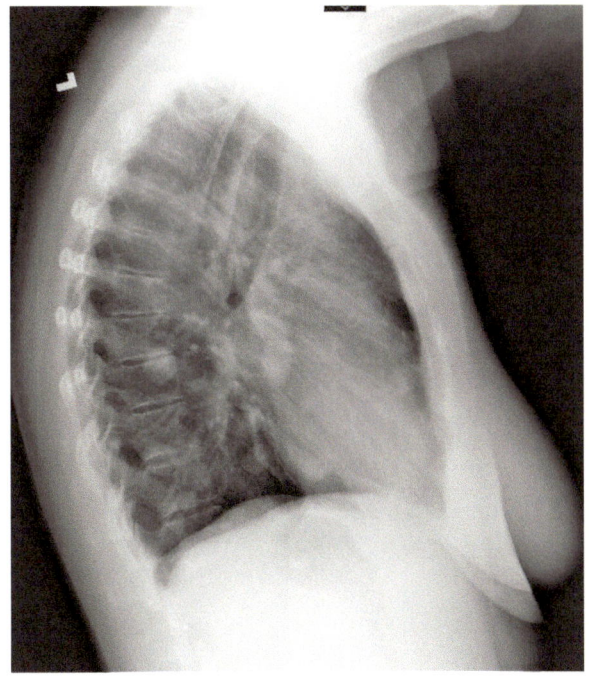

Fig. 4.8 CXR with *arrows* indicating the multiple nodules (*small arrows*) and mass (*large arrow*)

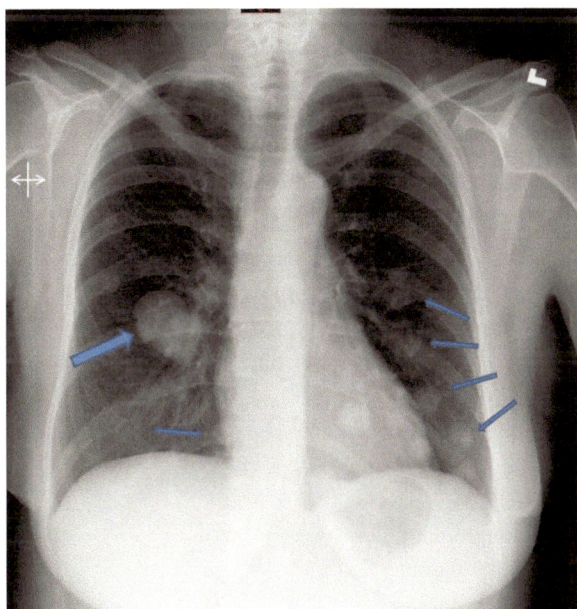

Fig. 4.9 PA showing large masses on *right*

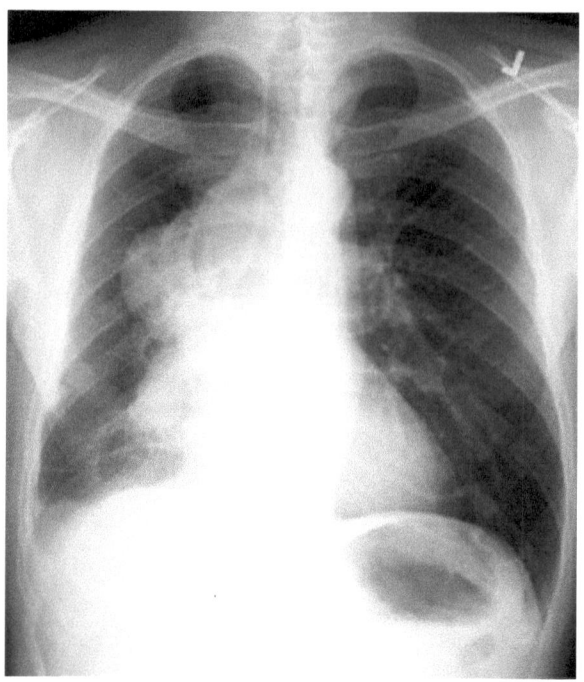

Radiological Signs

Approximately 20% of bronchial carcinoids arise peripherally, distal to the segmental bronchi. The majority of these neoplasms are of the atypical subtype. Both typical and atypical subtypes can be associated with hilar and mediastinal lymphadenopathy; hyperplasia results from repeated post-obstructive infections or metastasis. Local nodal metastasis is more common in atypical carcinoids.

Case 4.3

Figures 4.9–4.12 show multiple large masses.

Findings: Widening of mediastinum superiorly on the right. Opacity in the retrosternal clear space seen on the lateral, heterogeneously enhancing perihilar mass post IV contrast on CT.

Pattern: Mass.

Differential Diagnosis
- Malignancy
- Granulomatous
- Inflammation, other

Fig. 4.10 Lateral demonstrating large perihilar masses

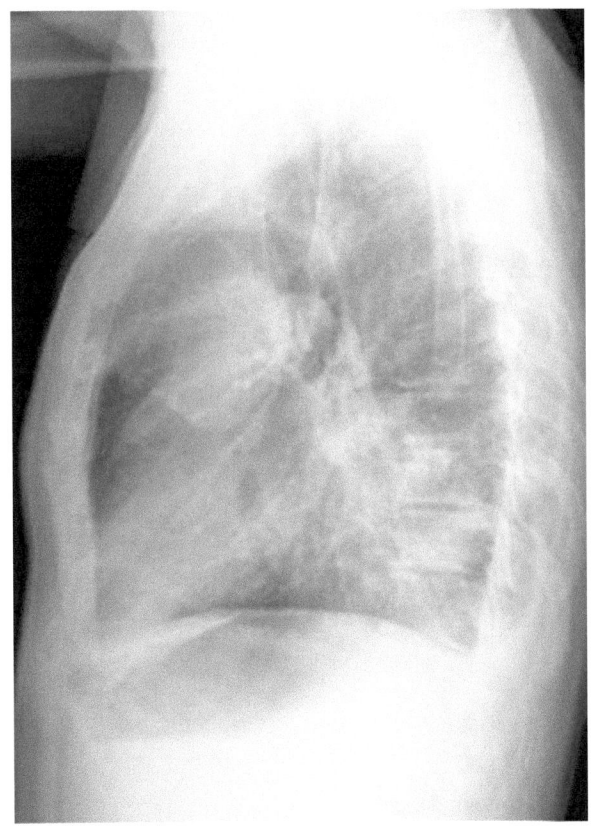

Fig. 4.11 Axial CT at level of carina (*C*) showing large heterogeneously enhancing mass (*M*) anteriolateral to ascending aorta (*A*) representing a bronchial carcinoid. There is also a pleural effusing noted on CT (*Eff*). Note also the descending aorta (*DA*), the left pulmonary artery (*LPA*)

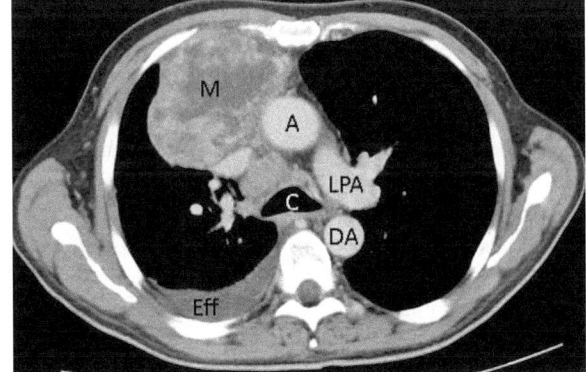

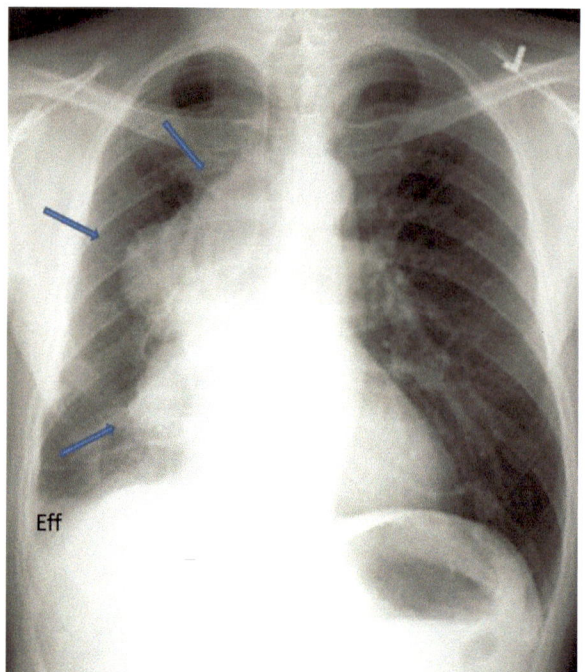

Fig. 4.12 PA again, with *arrows* highlighting masses. Also note blunting of the costophrenic angle on the *right* (*Eff*)

- Benign neoplasm
- Congenital

Based on location of masses in this case, extra-parenchymal considerations should include the anterior mediastinal mass differential (the 6 "Ts"). This particular case was lymphoma.

Granulomatous Disease

A granulomatous reaction in the chest usually produces nodules or small masses in the lungs. The earliest manifestations may be diffuse interstitial or mixed infiltration in the form of nodules consisting mainly of epithelioid macrophages and other inflammatory and immune cells.

Granulomatous conditions are classified here as either infectious or non-infectious for the purposes of findings and arriving at a reasonable differential.

Table 4.1 identifies some of the many and varied granulomatous mass (nodule) patterns that can be seen on CXR.

Table 4.1 Patterns and characteristics supporting granulomatous disease

Lung mass	Solitary pulmonary nodule
Radiological characteristics	
Homogenous soft tissue density	Soft tissue (or calcific) density less than 3 cm in diameter
Density greater than 3 cm in diameter (less than 3 cm is a nodule)	Distinct margins
Sharp margins	Oval or round
Masses do not respect fissures, however, may displace them	Consider metastasis
Granulomatous etiologies	
Granulomatous infections (Tuberculosis [TB], Histoplasmosis Blastomycosis)	Granulomas (often calcified)
Wegener's granuloma	Other infectious etiology
	Benign nodules
Lymphadenopathy	Cavity
Radiological characteristics	
Widening of mediastinum	Number: single or multiple (consider metastasis)
Polycyclic margin	Size: mm to cm
Clear space between heart and the nodal density with hilar nodes	Location: apices of lobes for TB, classical segments for aspiration
Extra-pleural sign with mediastinal nodes	Thickness of wall: thick, thin
Obliteration of silhouette based on location	Fluid level: consider abscess, fungous ball
Widening of carina with subcarinal nodes	Lumen: regular or irregular
	Associated findings
Granulomatous etiologies	
Granulomatous diseases	Wegener's granuloma
TB	Granulomatous infections, TB, Histoplasmosis
Sarcoidosis	See the "CAVITY" mnemonic
Histoplasmosis	
Silicosis	

Note: Consider neoplasia/metastasis with any mass

Note: you can use *CAVITY* as a mnemonic to help you remember the differential for cavitary lesions in the chest:

CAVITY:
C – Cancer, congenital, or acquired bullae
A – Abscess
V – Vasculitis
I – Infection (fungal, granulomatous)
T – Tuberculosis (TB)
Y – cYst (posttraumatic)

Fig. 4.13 CXR of infectious granulomatous disease

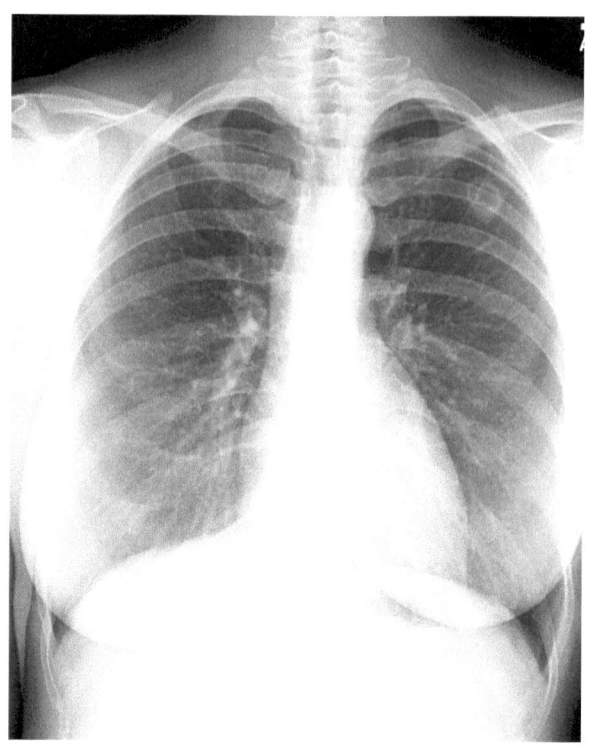

Infectious Granulomatous Disease

Infectious granulomatous diseases are frequently identified as nodules (or mass) on a CXR. This can happen with the following diseases.

- Tuberculosis
- Atypical mycobacterial diseases – especially Mycobacterium Avium-Intracellular (MAI)
- Fungal diseases
  - Coccidioidomycosis
  - Blastomycosis (North American and South American)
  - Cryptococcosis
  - Sporotrichosis
- Bacterial diseases, nocardiosis and/or actinomycosis

Case 4.4

The following case (Figs. 4.13 – 4.15) presents a 28-year-old female who had a CXR to monitor a preexisting lesion, though she was asymptomatic at the time of the CXR. She lived in central California.

Fig. 4.14 Lateral CXR of infectious granulomatous disease

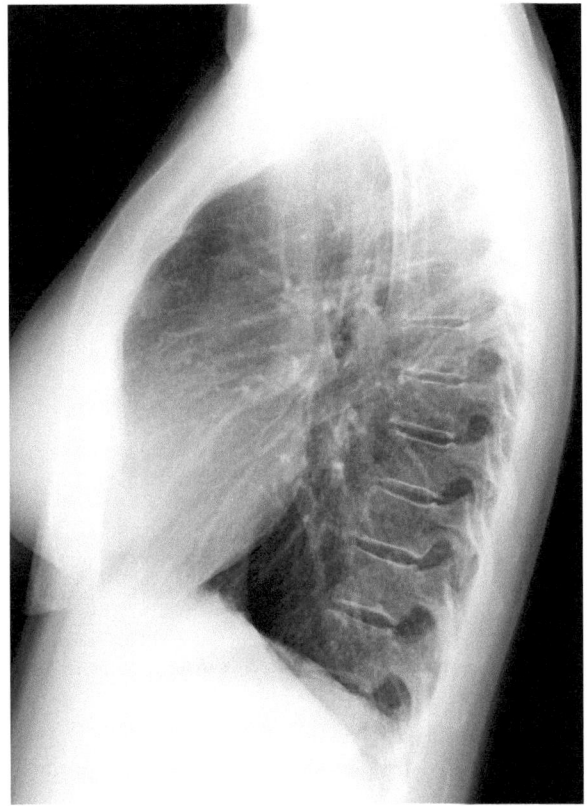

Findings: Opacity with central lucency in Left Upper Lobe posteriorly.
Pattern: Mass, cavitary.
Differential Diagnosis

Since cavitary, consider the CAVITARY mnemonic differential.
Wegener's granulomatosis can appear just like this.

The standard mass differential:
- Malignancy
- Granulomatous
- Inflammation
- Benign neoplasm
- Congenital

Diagnosis: Coccidiomycosis.
In this case, history helped narrow the diagnosis further, as the patient grew up in the San Joaquin River valley: Coccidiomycosis is also known as San Joaquin Valley Fever.
Signs: Fever, cervical adenopathy, skin lesions, pleural effusion, friction rub, pulmonary rales.

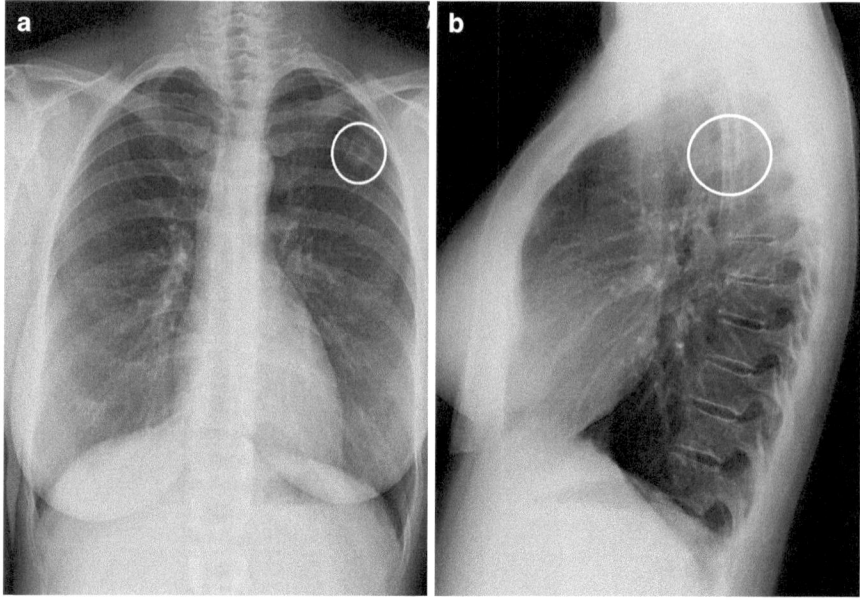

Fig. 4.15 (a) PA with *circle* highlighting cavitary (*coin*) lesion representing coccidiomycosis. Note suggestion of air-fluid level. (b) Lateral showing subtle cavity (*due to overlying shoulders*) lesion

Symptoms: Include chills, weight loss, productive cough, chest pain, and arthralgias.

Diagnostic tests: Include sputum smear (KOH test), sputum culture, serology, CXR, and the Coccidioidin/Spherulin skin test.

Treatment: The acute disease almost always goes away without treatment. Bed rest and treatment of flu-like symptoms until fever disappears may be recommended. Disseminated or severe disease should be treated with amphotericin B, ketoconazole, fluconazole, or itraconazole.

Non-infectious Granulomatous Disease

The following are non-infectious granulomatous conditions:

- Sarcoidosis
- Hypersensitivity Pneumonitis (HP)
- Vasculitis-granulomatosis diseases
  - Wegener's
  - Lymphocytic
  - Bronchocentric allergic (Churg–Strauss)
- Langerhans granulomatosis (eosinophilic granuloma, histiocytosis) (LCG)

Fig. 4.16 Nocardia lung infection manifesting as multiple lung nodules. Also note ground-glass opacities in right lung

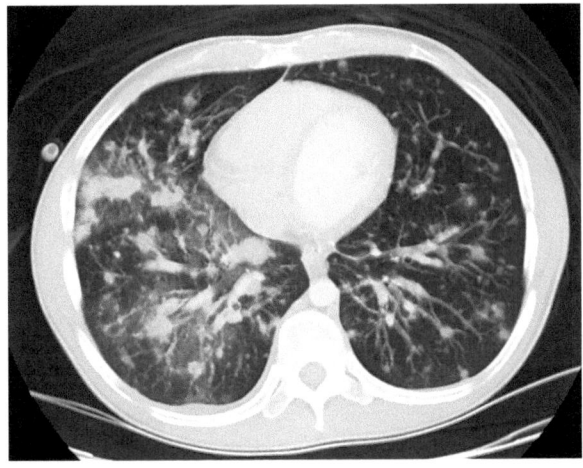

Inflammation (Non-granulomatous)

Many processes can resemble a mass and be appropriately classified (from a finding perspective) into the mass category. The importance is deriving a conclusion based on findings, patterns, and the clinical third dimension.

An example of inflammatory mass would be an abscess. This can appear like the previous case of a cavitary lesion (coccidiomycosis case).

Another example would be infection that manifests as multiple nodules or masses. See Fig. 4.16 for a case of *Nocardia* lung infection manifesting as multiple lung nodules.

Benign Neoplasm

A benign tumor takes on the shape of a well-defined opacity, whereas a malignant tumor has more spiculated and irregular margins.

Hamartoma

Hamartomas are common benign neoplasms, of which 90% are found in the lung. Hamartomas make up 5% of all solitary lung nodules. They have the following characteristics.

They frequently contain cartilage with fibrous connective tissue and various amounts of fat, smooth muscle, and seromucous glands.

Approximately 30% contain calcium, usually of the "popcorn" variety.

They are seen most commonly in the fourth and fifth decades of life.

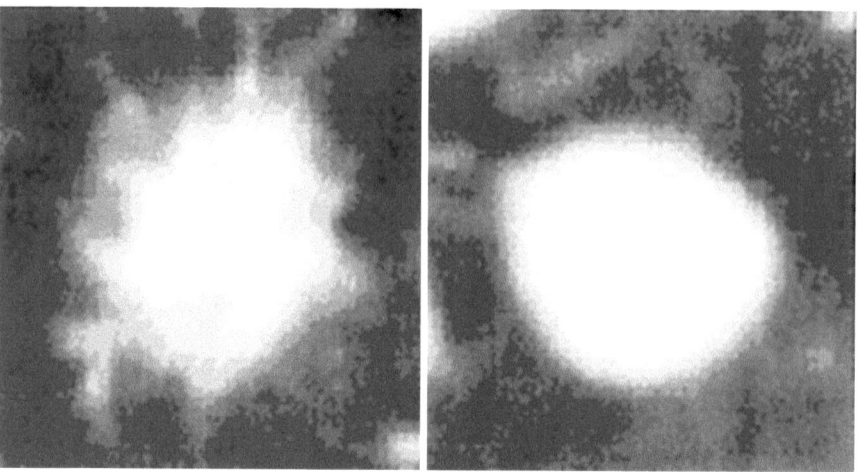

Fig. 4.17 The malignant mass (*left*) is spiculated and the benign mass (*right*) has smooth margins

Fig. 4.18 This AP CXR
demonstrates a well-
circumscribed calcified
rounded/lobulated nodule
near right cardiac border

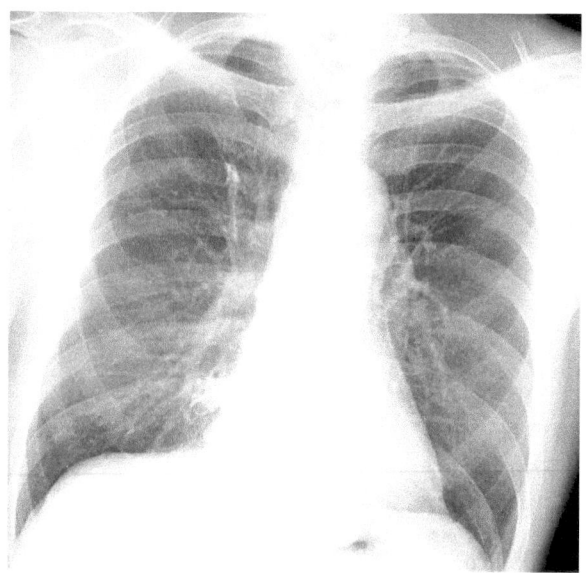

Case 4.6

Figures 4.18 and 4.19 are examples of a hamartoma.

Findings: Popcorn-like calcification in right lung field near right heart border. CT
verifies location in right middle lobe and further characterizes as a popcorn-shaped
calcification. A calcified granuloma is incidentally seen in the right upper lung field
on the CXR.

Fig. 4.19 CT of same patient showing calcification in RML; note the shape resembles popcorn, compatible with hamartoma

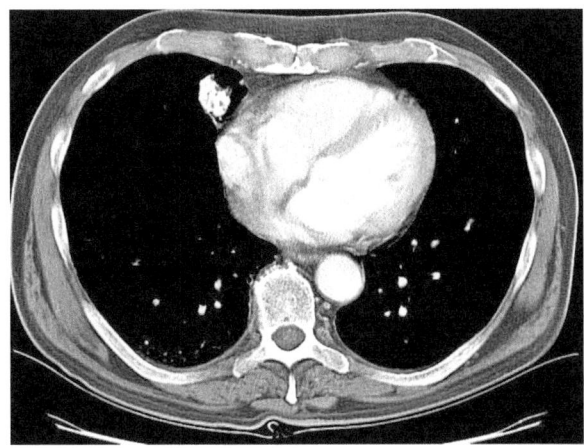

Pattern: Mass (nodule).

Differential Diagnosis: This finding is nearly characteristic of benign neoplasm, specifically hamartoma. Granuloma is less of a consideration since the nodule in this case is irregularly calcified. Of the general mass differential, inflammation, congenital, and malignancy are less likely.

Congenital Abnormality

Pulmonary Arteriovenous Malformations

Certain congenital conditions such as **Pulmonary Arteriovenous Malformations** can resemble mass and therefore satisfy the mass category.

Case 4.7

An example is shown below with several mass-like structures seen on the initial CXR.

Findings: Multiple focal opacities seen bilaterally, sparing the apicies.

Pattern: Mass, multiple.

Differential Diagnosis
- Malignancy
- Granulomatous
- Inflammation, other
- Benign neoplasm
- Congenital

Fig. 4.20 PA CXR demonstrating multiple nodules and masses (*within dotted ovals*)

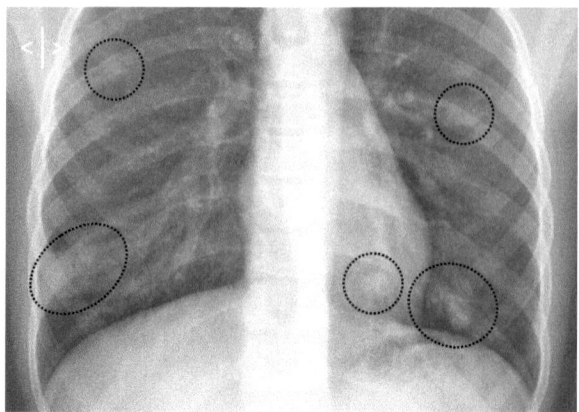

Fig. 4.21 CT demonstrating feeding and draining vessels, confirming AVM

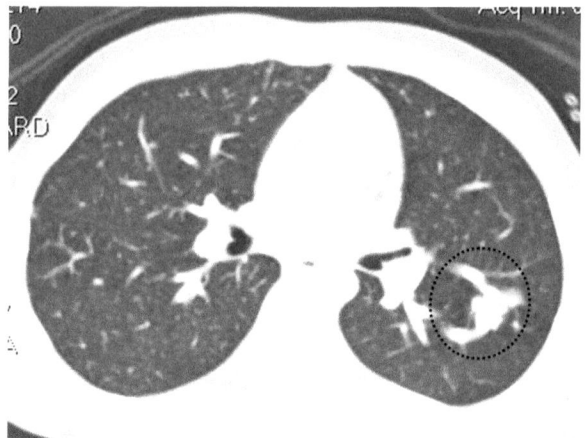

Malignancy and congenital were highest on the differential due to multiplicity. CT was obtained (below) confirming multiple pulmonary arteriovenous malformations (AVM) in the lung.

Pulmonary AVMs are abnormal connections between the pulmonary arteries and veins. They are single in 65% of the cases, multiple in 35%. They are twice as common in women as in men, and the majority are congenital and are found in the lower lobes. Significantly, nearly 70% are associated with Hereditary Hemorrhagic Telangiectasia (Osler-Weber-Rendu disease), an autosomal dominant condition involving multiple AVMs in the brain, lung, skin, and liver.

Consolidation

Consolidation is defined as alveolar space that contains the fluid instead of air. In pneumonia, consolidation results when an infected lung passes from an aerated collapsible condition to one of airless solid consistency through the accumulation of exudates in the alveoli and adjoining ducts.

Fig. 4.22 Drawing of pulmonary alveoli in the secondary pulmonary lobule (Image courtesy of Mariana Ruiz Villarreal). Consolidation results when the alveoli fill with pus and is also referred to as "air-space opacities"

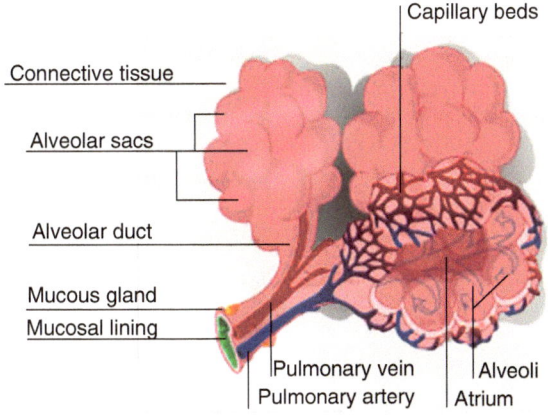

Fig. 4.23 This is an example RML consolidation abutting the horizontal fissure superiorly. This demonstrates how pneumonia respects fissures and how the margin can be sharp, sometimes resembling a mass

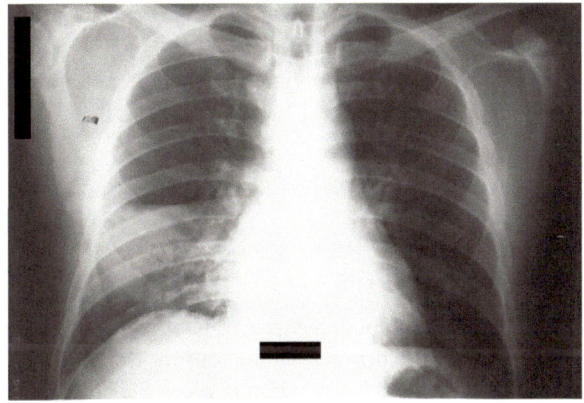

Consolidation may be mimicked by alveolar collapse, as in an airway obstruction, but is not a collapse of the alveola; rather, it is a filling of the alveolar spaces with a fluid. The fluid can be pulmonary edema, inflammatory exudates, pus, inhaled water, or blood.

Consolidative Radiological Findings/Distribution

Consolidative radiological signs include:

- Fluffy, cloud-like, coalescent opacities.
- Complete air bronchograms seen through the opacity.
- Obliterates pulmonary vasculature.
- There can be sharp edges when limited by fissures or pleura (see Fig. 4.23).

  Distribution: Lobar (in pneumonia), diffuse (as in edema)
  Differentiates from "ground glass" (not SOLID)

Fig. 4.24 Right lower lung field opacification. Note that the right heart border and right hemidiaphragm are obliterated, indicating RML and RLL consolidations

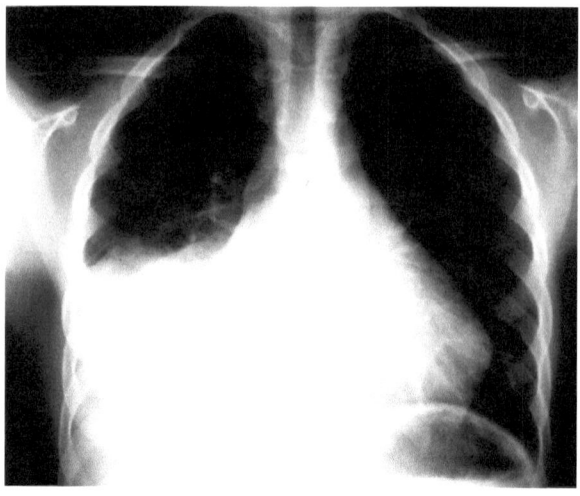

Consolidation may be caused by (differential):

- Hemorrhage – Blood
- Exudate – Pus
- Transudate – Water
- Secretions – Protein
- Malignancy – Cells

The mantra: "blood, pus, water, protein, cells" helps students and residents recall the consolidative differential and ensure it is understood and communicated. Also remember that conSOLIDation is more SOLID than ground glass opacities or airway pattern.

Consolidative Model

The following case/figures depict a model analogous to radiological findings of consolidation.

In the following PA and lateral CXR (Fig. 4.24 and 4.25), note the silhouette sign obscuring the right cardiac silhouette (right atrium) and right hemidiaphragm that help further localize the process. Also note the air bronchograms best seen on the lateral. There is a positive spine sign in that the spine does not get darker inferiorly as it should, indicating overlying density in the lower lobe consolidation.

Considering the case presented above, look at the common visual illusion below that can look either like two white faces (facing each other) or one central black vase.

This is presented to consider the air bronchogram, with the air as the exception in a predominantly dense consolidation. This is in contrast to the tram tracks that are two densities surrounding the bronchus in bronchiectasis, with the density as the exception to the predominant airway. These two concepts are often confused by

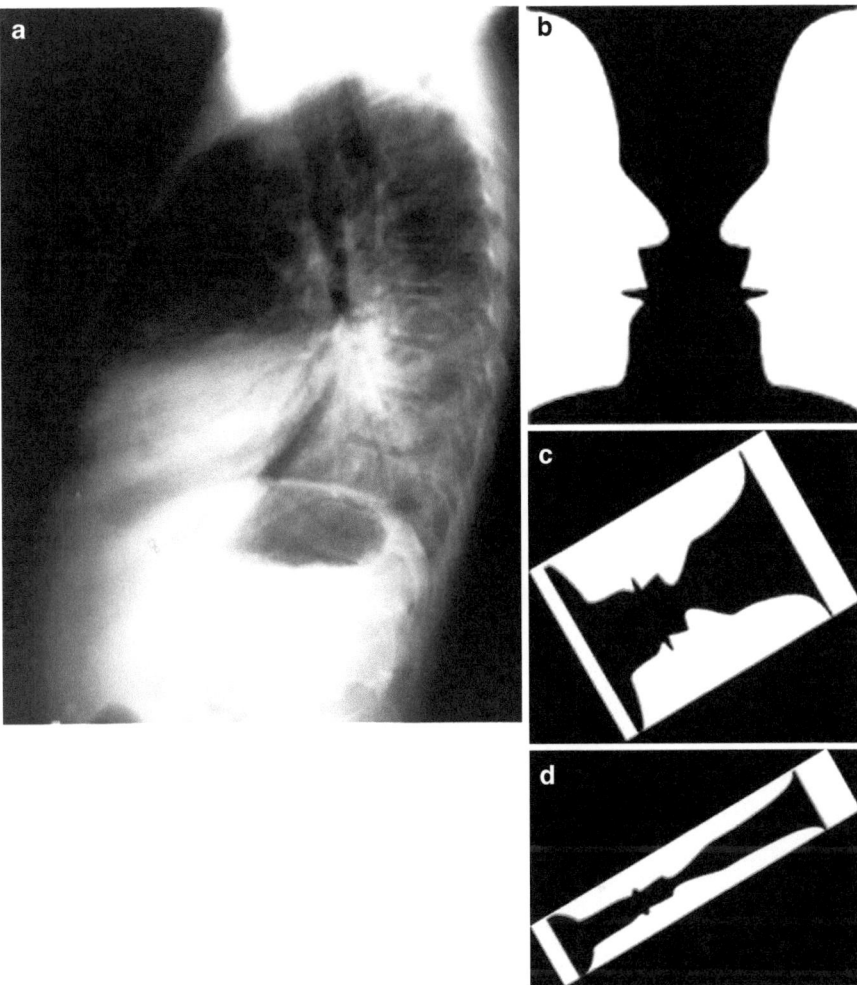

Fig. 4.25 Consolidative pattern, lateral view (**a**). Note positive spine sign, lucencies representing air-bronchograms and obliteration of right hemidiaphragm. The face-vase illusion (**b**) and tilted image (**c**) and squeezed (**d**) to simulate an air-bronchogram. See Fig. 4.26 for superimposed graphic on X-ray (Original image courtesy of S. Lehar. Manipulated versions of image created by USUHS ETI Support Office)

the beginning radiology student, hence are presented together to contrast these two very different entities.

Figure 4.26b depicts the popular faces and vase illusion and purposely narrowed to represent air as the exception as an analog to the air bronchogram within a consolidation, such as this case.

The following case again demonstrates air bronchograms with another analogy (see Fig. 4.2) [5].

The left lower lung field in this 53 year old contains a "complete air bronchogram," meaning the tubular lucency extends from hilum to periphery. The right lower lung shows a less obvious air bronchogram exiting the hilum inferiorly.

Fig. 4.26 Air as the
exception in the air
bronchogram with
superimposed just *above*,
highlighting the air
bronchogram concept.
The air-bronchograms are
parallel to the illusion, just
below it

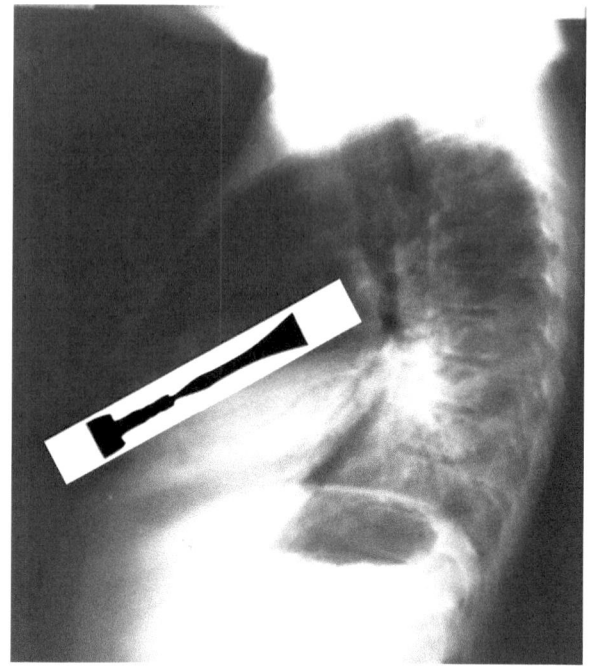

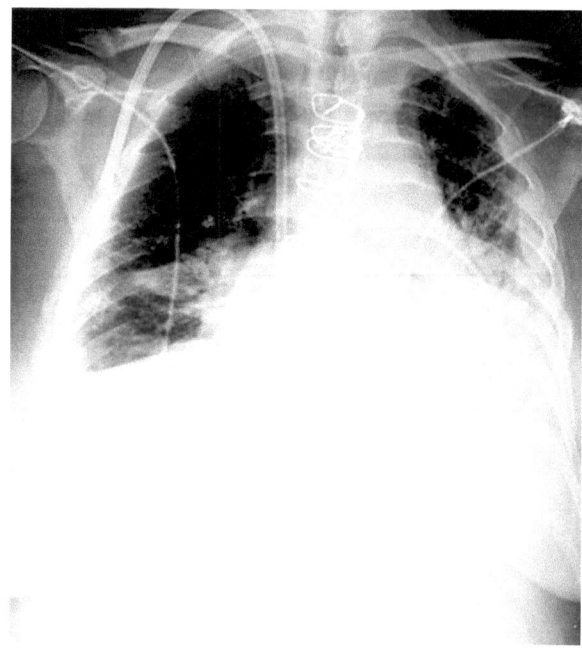

Fig. 4.27 Note the air
bronchograms (lucencies in
retrocardiac density) in the
left lower lung field
representing consolidation

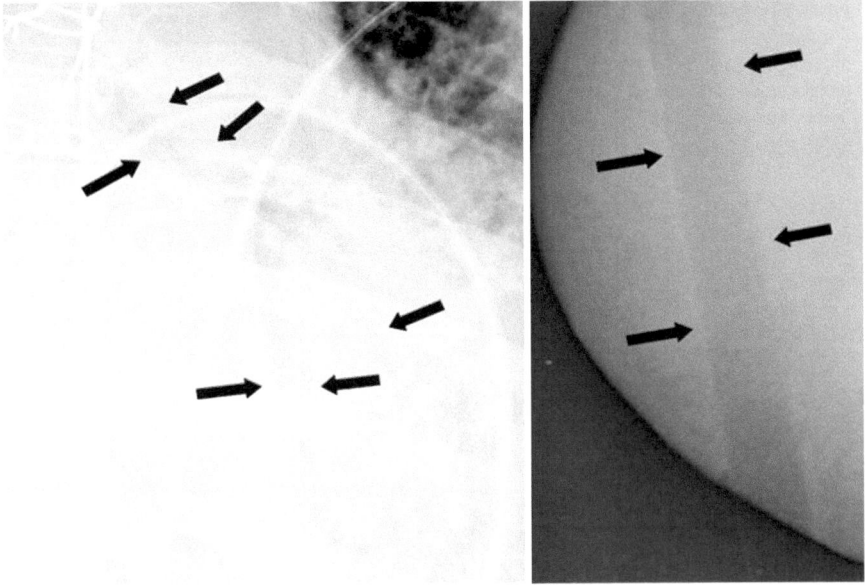

Fig. 4.28 Close-up of air bronchogram (*left*); close-up of air bronchogram analog created in an apple with a straw (*right*). See Fig. 4.29 for how this image was created

Figure 4.28 provides a magnified view of the above CXR alongside of an X-Ray of an apple with a straw through it (see Fig. 4.29 for experiment setup) that resembles an air bronchogram.

See also the Bronchial Wall Thickening Model in the airway section of this chapter.

Blood (Hemorrhage)

Case 4.8

Blunt force to lung tissue causes bruising as force does in many other soft tissue analogs. See Fig. 4.30 for an example of a contusion of the lung manifesting as a consolidation. This patient suffered a blast injury to the right side.

Findings: Contused right lung peripherally (just below proximal port of chest tube). Other findings include right hemopneumothorax, chest tube, metallic fragment from blast.

Pattern: Consolidation.

Differential Diagnosis: Lung contusion.

Diagnosis: Right lung contusion; in addition, traumatic hemopneumothorax (note the air-fluid level).

Fig. 4.29 Apple with straw
through it on X-ray plate
to create figure 4.28
(right image). The air
in the straw contrasted
the surrounding apple

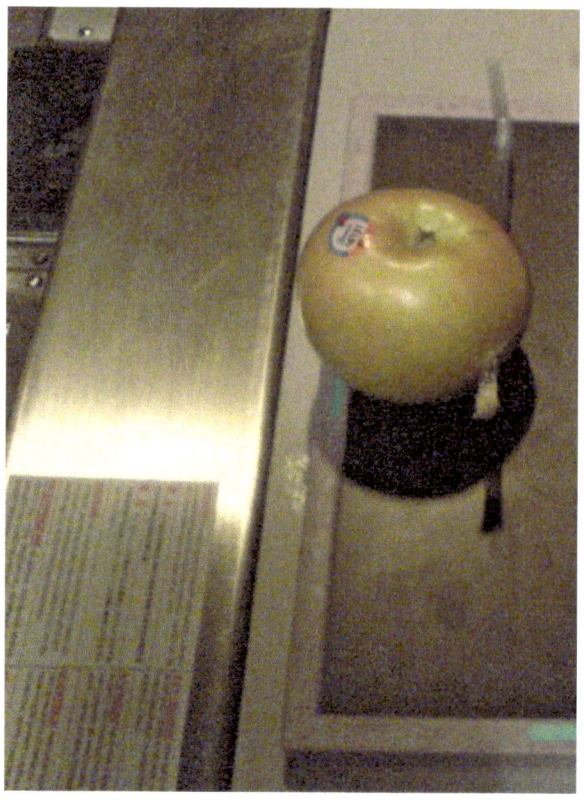

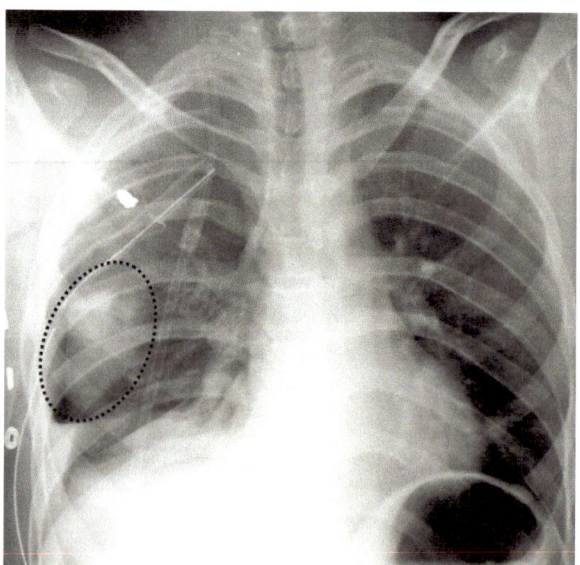

Fig. 4.30 Consolidation
representing hemorrhage
(*density highlighted by dotted
oval*). Additionally noted is
chest tube, blast fragment,
and hydropneumothorax
(*air-fluid level*)

Fig. 4.31 Opacification of the right upper lung field representing a consolidation pattern in bacterial pneumonia in the RUL. Location is confirmed by horizontal fissure inferiorly on the PA and lateral, and the major fissure on the lateral

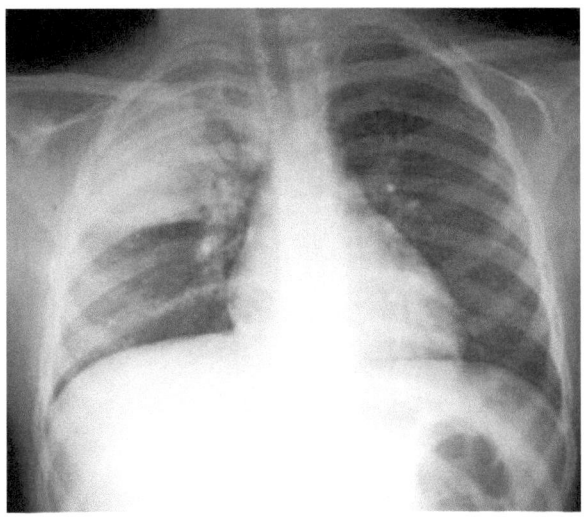

Pus (Exudate)

Pus from a variety of infections can cause pneumonia. Pneumonia generally respects lobes; hence distribution is lobar or multilobar. However, atypical pneumonia may be diffuse and bilateral.

Some pneumonias originate in the lung periphery where the *Streptococcus pneumoniae* reaches the lung via the airway. In lower right lobe pneumonia especially, aspiration should be considered since the right mainstem bronchus and bronchus intermedius are more vertical than on the left.

Bacterial Pneumonia
- Is most commonly caused by *Streptococcus pneumoniae*
- May present with mild to severe symptoms, including shaking chills, chattering teeth, severe chest pain, and a cough productive of rust-colored or greenish sputum
- May be febrile, diaphoretic, tachypneic, dyspneic, and/or cyanotic

Case 4.9

Figures 4.31 and 4.32 depict lobar consolidation in the RUL, with fissures limiting extension.

Findings
RUL: Large area of airspace opacification on the frontal view has both major and minor fissures as its inferior border. The lateral view demonstrates nicely the fissures of the right lung. Both RML and RLL remain well aerated.

Pattern: Consolidation.
Differential Diagnosis: Bacterial Lobar Pneumonia.

Fig. 4.32 Lobar
consolidation pattern
on lateral. Note the airspace
opacity limited inferiorly by
the minor fissue anteriorly
and the major fissure
posteriorly

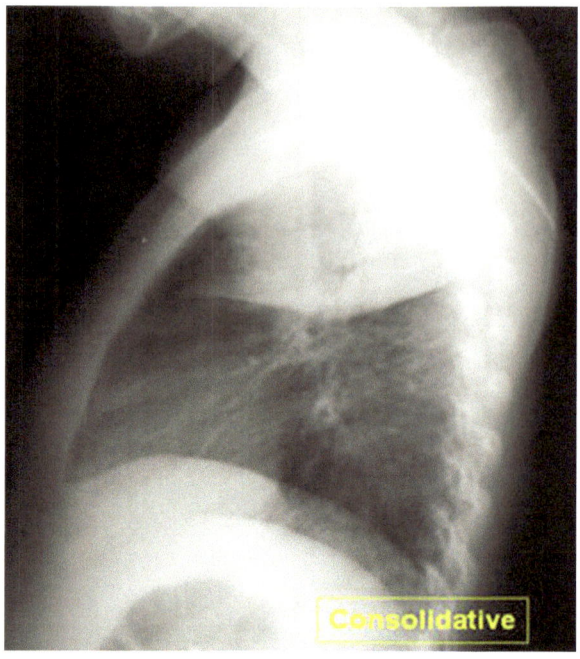

Case 4.10

In some cases, a consolidation can resemble a mass, as shown on the CXR in this case. Additionally, this case demonstrates radiopaque markers that attempt to show degree of inclination (however, unsuccessfully). Lastly, this AP portable is an example of a rotated right projection. (Note the clavicles are to the right of the spine.)

Findings: RUL opacity bordering minor fissure inferiorly, however, maintains fluffy superior margin.

Pattern: Consolidation.

Note: Mass could also be considered, however, since abutment to horizontal fissure inferiorly gives the impression of mass (such as malignancy). A follow-up CXR documenting the resolution is paramount to rule out mass in cases like this.

Differential Diagnosis: Pneumonia, loculated fluid in horizontal fissure (pseudomass); mass differential can be considered until ruled out by CT or follow-up CXRs.

Diagnosis: RUL bacterial lobar pneumonia, confirmed by resolution with antibiotics and follow-up CXR.

Note the small ball bearings (BBs) in the left marker indicating an upright projection. Experience with these, however, demonstrates that the BBs fall to this location starting at 30° of inclination. Work is being done to achieve higher accuracy (discussed in the pleural section of this book).

Fig. 4.33 Right upper lobe pneumonia; again limited inferiorly by the horizontal fissure, in this case making it resemble a mass

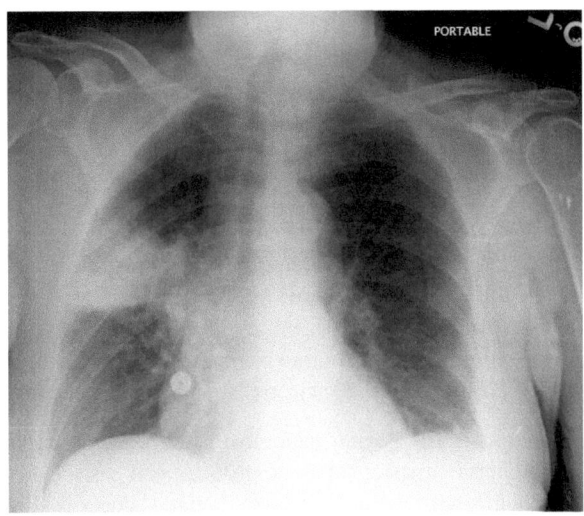

Fig. 4.34 Note the medial clavicles (*outlined in black*) and the orientation relative to the vertebral spinous processes (*outlined in teardrop shapes*). This indicates the patient is rotated toward their *right*

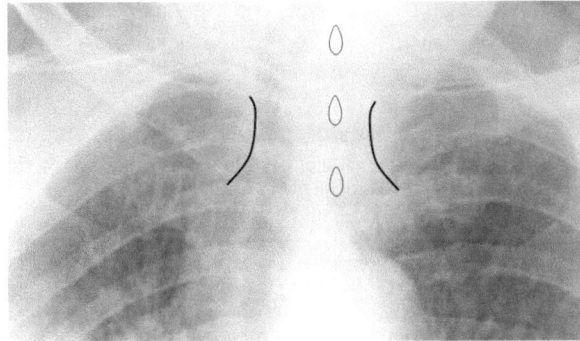

Water (Transudate)

Water can cause congestion and appear as airspace opacities/consolidation. See examples below for a transudate manifesting as a consolidation.

Pulmonary Edema

Pulmonary edema is not a disease by itself; it represents accumulation of fluid in extravascular lung from underlying process. We can divide it into four main categories based on pathophysiology.

1. *Increase hydrostatic pressure edema*: There are two phases: interstitial edema and alveolar edema. This is most commonly seen in left-sided heart failure in the ICU and ER. The interstitial phase often includes peribronchial cuffing and septal lines. The alveolar phase often includes batwing airspace opacities.

2. *Permeability edema with diffuse alveolar damage*: There are several precipitating factors unrelated to cardiac insufficiency. Pulmonary or extrapulmonary ARDS is the most severe and has three overlapping stages.
   - *Exudative stage*: Interstitial edema resulting in alveolar filling (hence it skips the interstitial pattern).
   - *Proliferative stage*: Inhomogeneous ground-glass opacities (can have a mixture of all three in this stage).
   - *Fibrotic stage*: Cystic areas may be seen and can cause pneumothorax.

3. *Permeability edema without diffuse alveolar damage*: Often results in patchy, bilateral airspace opacities, ill-defined vessels, peribronchial cuffing. Unlike edema with diffuse alveolar damage, these findings can reverse. It is seen in heroin-induced pulmonary edema or following the administration of cytokines and in high-altitude pulmonary edema.

4. *Mixed edema*: This is generally an airspace opacification finding, depending on etiology (neurogenic, reperfusion, status post lung, transplant, re-expansion, post pneumonectomy, post reduction, air embolism).

Findings often vary in daily ICU CXRs, helping narrow differential to edema in that infection does not usually clear within a day or two (for example).

Case 4.11

This first case is a young male suffering from an MI. Figures 4.35 and 4.36 demonstrate a fast transition from a normal CXR to an abnormal diffuse airspace process.

Findings: Bilateral and diffuse fluffy/patchy airspace and reticulo-nodular opacities. Also, ET tube tip is well above the carina (note measurement, 5.7 cm) and enteric tube in stomach.

Pattern: Consolidation, diffuse bilaterally. One could consider ground glass and reticulo-nodular (interstitial) pattern.

Differential Diagnosis: Acute (or Adult) Respiratory Distress Syndrome (ARDS), pulmonary edema (although small heart). The reason "pus" is not as highly considered is the acuteness of the process and the lack of fever or other infectious symptoms before the arrest. Also, pneumonias typically respect fissures and not immediately diffuse. The same goes for "cells" differential because this is a young patient who had a normal CXR hours before.

Diagnosis: Acute respiratory failure can occur two basic ways: failure of respiratory pump to deliver adequate oxygen to healthy lungs (neurogenic), or failure of

Fig. 4.35 The first portable
AP projection fails to
demonstrate airspace
opacities or other abnormality
(*normal CXR*)

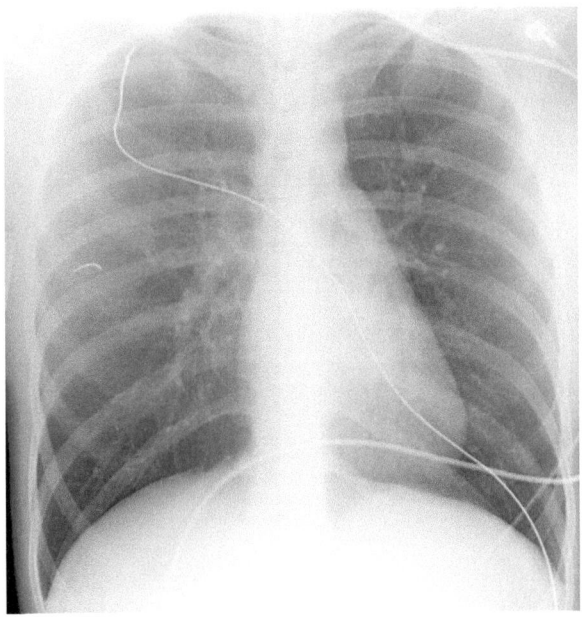

Fig. 4.36 This follow-up
portable CXR (on the same
patient) was obtained a few
hours later in the ICU after
the patient required
ventilatory support. Note the
diffuse patchy airspace
opacities representing edema
(transudate)

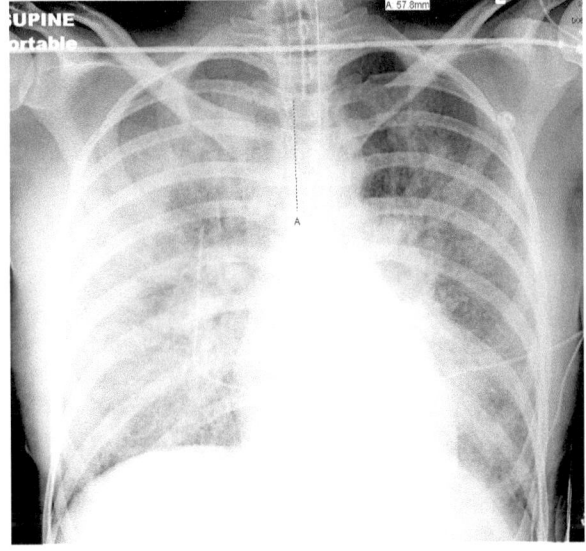

damaged lungs to manage gas exchange. Diffusely damaged lungs are characteristic
of ARDS, which consists of acute respiratory distress, progressive hypoxemia
refractory to oxygen administration, increasing lung stiffness, and diffuse radiographic lung opacification.

Fig. 4.37 Diffuse airspace opacities (consolidative pattern) caused by blast injury

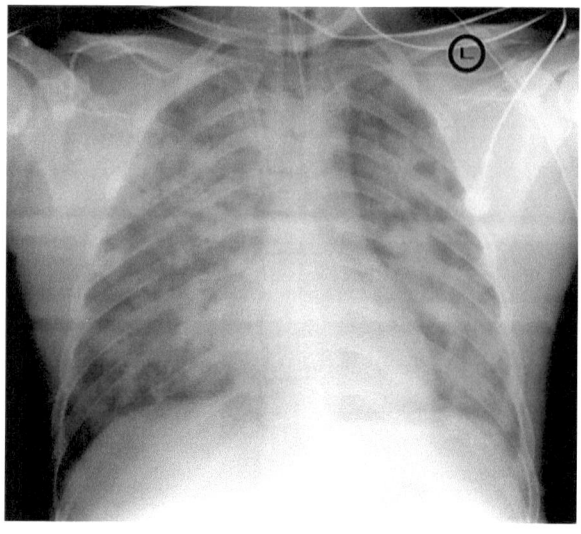

Case 4.12

The young soldier in Fig. 4.37 was exposed to a blast.

Findings: Bilateral and diffuse fluffy/patchy opacities. Also, ET well above carina, right and left central line tips in SVC, enteric tube in stomach.

Pattern: Consolidation, diffuse, patchy.

Differential Diagnosis: Secondary to (or concomitant with) ARDS.

Diagnosis: ARDS. Note: There remains some debate as to mechanisms of blast lung injury; however, from a clinical standpoint, this patient (as many post-blast patients) was diagnosed with ARDS before evacuation out of the combat zone.

Protein (Secretions)

Mucous protein can plug alveoli from a number of injuries and diseases, including Pulmonary Alveolar Proteinosis (PAP), shown in the case below. Keep in mind that this is a findings-based approach, and this same diagnostic category can be found through the interstitial pathway (similar to edema).

Case 4.13 (see Figs. 4.38 and 4.39)

Findings: Bilateral diffuse fluffy/ patchy airspace opacities.
Pattern: Consolidation (could also be categorized as interstitial).
Differential Diagnosis: ARDS, PAP, aspiration, and less likely interstitial considerations.
Diagnosis: PAP. CT shows crazy paving (see Fig. 4.39).

Fig. 4.38 Portable CXR done in ICU demonstrating diffuse patchy airspace opacities. Additionally there are the following tubes/lines: ET tube in trachea above carina, feeding tube in stomach, two left chest tubes, PICC line at junction of left brachycephalic and SVC

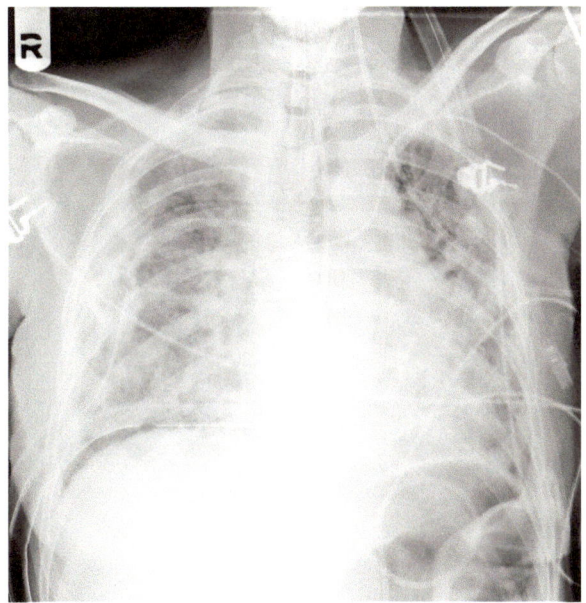

Fig. 4.39 CT of same patient demonstrating "crazy paving" in RML and RLL (*thin arrows on patient's right*) and bronchiectasis within consolidated LLL (*wide arrow on patient's left*)

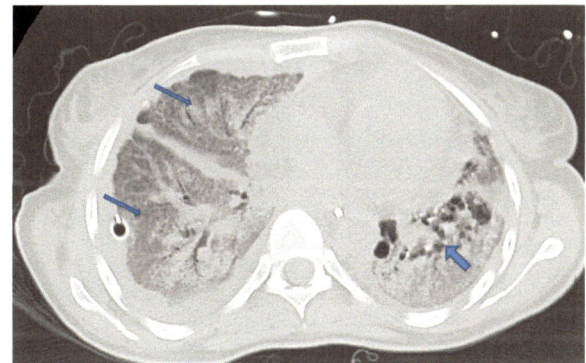

Cells (Malignancy)

Bronchoalveolar cell carcinoma (BAC), Kaposi's sarcoma, and lymphoma can display as a consolidative pseudo-mass.

Figure 4.40 demonstrate perihilar consolidations in a child with Kaposi's sarcoma.

Interstitial

Chest X-Rays showing interstitial markings include a large variety of abnormal processes including edema, inflammation, disease, and environmental exposure.

Fig. 4.40 (**a**) PA and (**b**)
lateral CXR demonstrating
irregular perihilar patchy
consolidations partially
obliterating vasculature and
right heart border in this
patient with Kaposi's
sarcoma

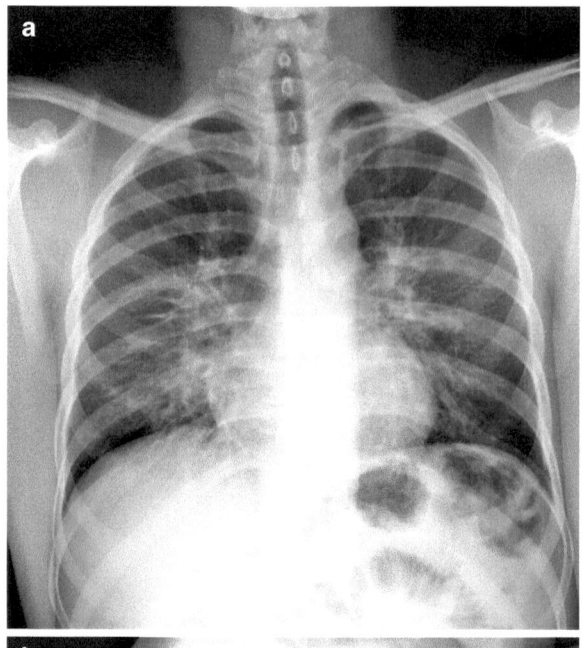
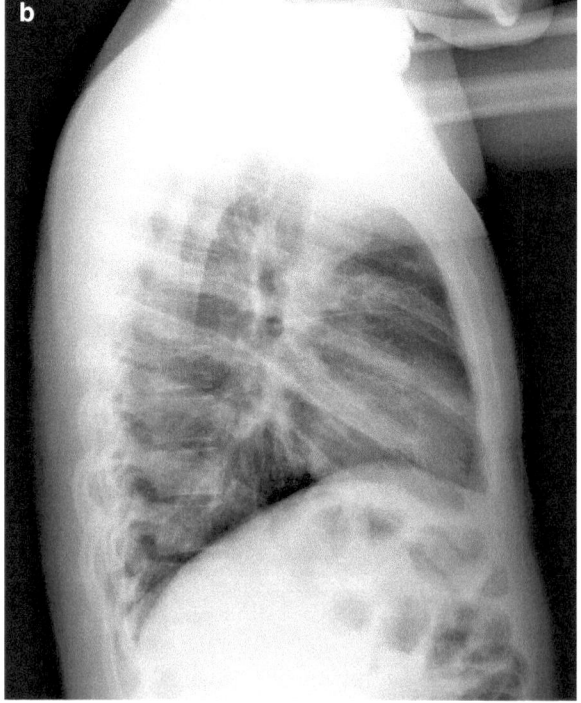

Fig. 4.41 End-stage "Honeycomb" lung (Image courtesy of Ed Uthman, M.D.)

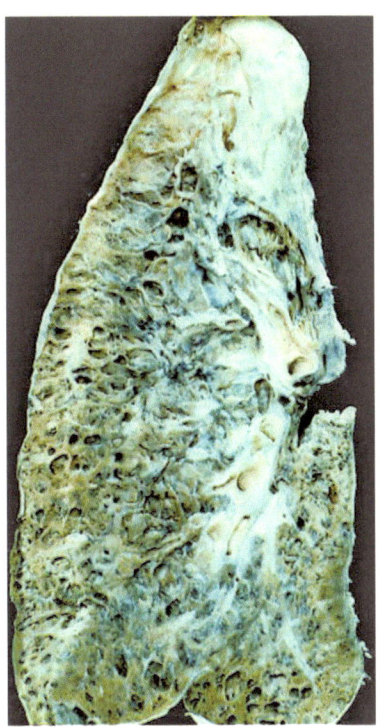

Interstitial markings appear on CXR and CT due to changes affecting the inter-stitium of the lung.

The composition of the pulmonary interstitium includes the:

- Alveolar walls, septi, and the connective tissue surrounding bronchi and vessels (peribronchial and perivascular spaces).
  Mechanisms of infiltration include:
- Thickening of lung interstices
- Architectural destruction of interstitium (honeycomb or "end-stage" lung)

Interstitial pattern includes lines, dots, and/or holes (any combination of the three) as opposed to the fluffy opacities seen with consolidation. Keep in mind there can be mixed patterns with consolidation, airway, mass, or vascular. On CT, ground glass is another finding in interstitial pattern.

An example of a disease that would produce an interstitial pattern, in this case, lines and holes (honeycomb pattern). Figure 4.41 is a gross specimen lung from a patient who had end-stage lung disease.

Fig. 4.42 CT showing
honeycomb lucencies in
upper lobes (*anteriorly* and
peripherally) bilaterally
(stacked lucencies with
bordering interstitial lines)

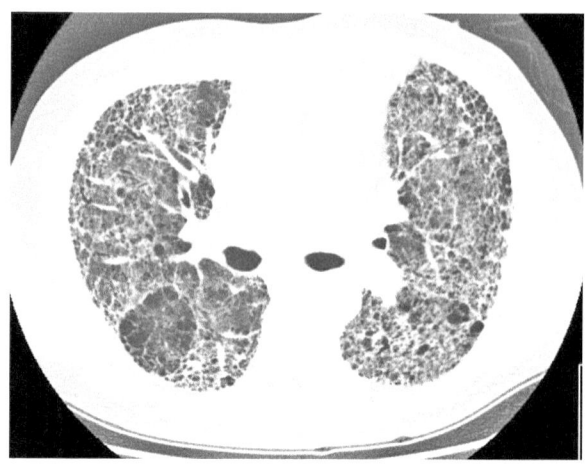

Radiological Signs

Interstitial markings can manifest in three basic forms on the CXR, and each form
has its own differential diagnosis.

Linear form (*lines*): Reticulations (lines in all directions, not just the branching
vessels) and septal lines (Kerley lines).

Nodular form (*dots*): Small, sharp, numerous, evenly distributed, uniform (especially uniform in shape) nodules.

Destructive form (*holes*): Peripheral, irregular cyst formation.

Linear Form: Lines

Linear Interstitial diseases include the following processes (pathologic types of the
linear form).

L – Lymphangitic spread/metastases
I – Inflammation, Infection
F – Fibrosis
E – Edema

You can use LIFE-lines (like the lines around a boat) as a mnemonic to help you
remember this list.

Case 4.14

Figures 4.43 and 4.44 show a CXR of a patient with lymphangitic spread, showing
lines running in all directions, followed by a CT used as an example of septal lines.

Findings: Diffuse lines distributed throughout lungs bilaterally.
Pattern: Interstitial, specifically lines (reticulations).

Differential diagnosis
L – Lymphangitic metastases (the diagnosis in this case)
I – Inflammation including infection
F – Fibrosis (less likely in this case due to pattern characteristics)
E – Edema (again less likely due to pattern characteristics, distribution)

To help differentiate interstitial lines in this case with normal tapering vasculature using an analogy with tree branching, see Fig. 4.43b comparing to normal left lower lung field.

In Figs. 4.44 – 4.46, you can see how in a CT of lymphangitic spread (here, the same case shown above), lines appear between vessels, like they do in a reticulated giraffe.

Figures 4.47 and 4.48 present another example of a CXR with an interstitial (specifically lines) pattern. This example shows Kerley lines in the LLL peripherally from interstitial edema.

Nodular Form: Dots

Nodules should be differentiated from normal vessels on-end before categorizing in the nodular pattern. See related information on the Mass Considerations at the beginning of this chapter.

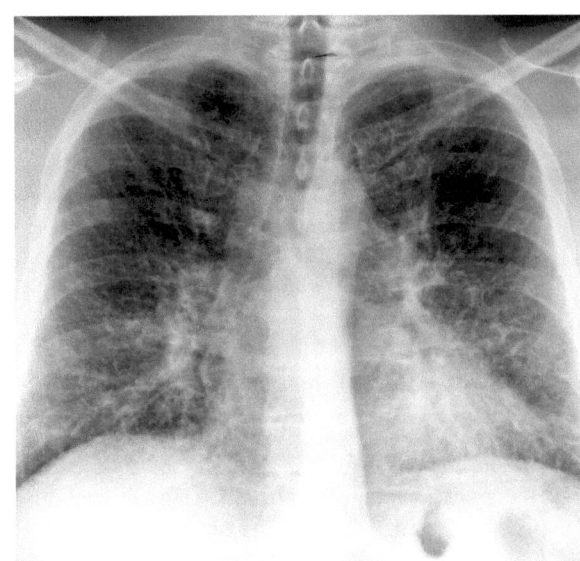

Fig. 4.43a Case of lymphangitic spread, showing diffuse lines (*all directions, crossing and obscuring vasculature*) throughout the lungs bilaterally

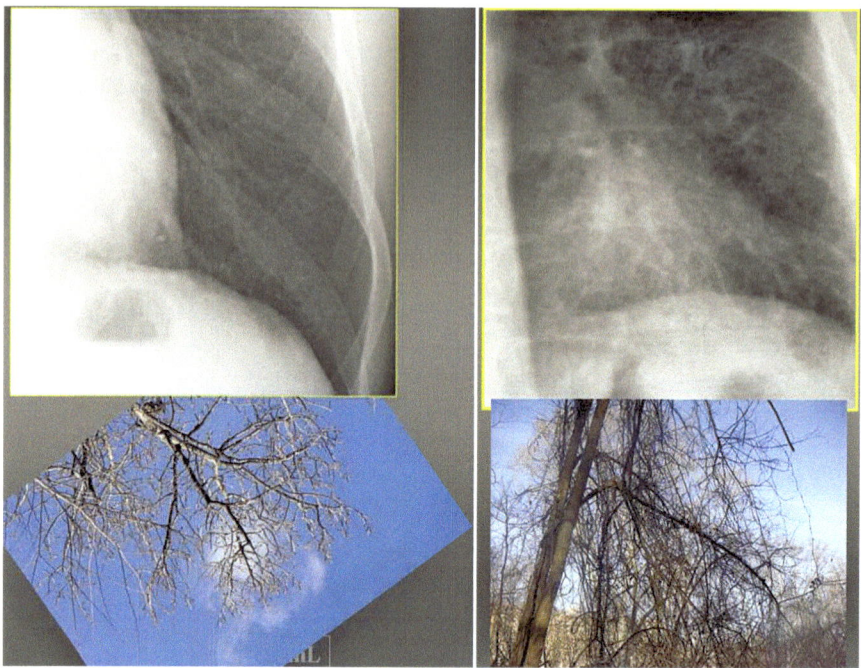

Fig. 4.43b Compare the normal tapering vessels on CXR (*left images*) similar to branching of trees to the crossing lines in all directions in our patient (*right images*). Note the crossing of lines is similar to how cudzu vines cross the normal tree branching, causing lines in all directions

Fig. 4.44 Lymphangitic spread on CT

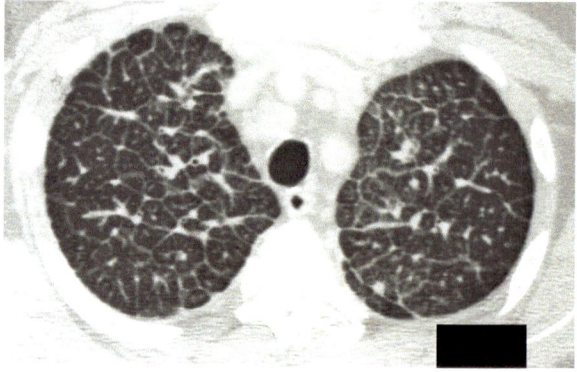

Processes resulting in nodular interstitial patterns include the following: Remember HGP for this differential (it somehow has a ring to it).

- Granulomatous diseases
- Hematogenous spread of malignancy, miliary disease, lymphocytic interstitial pneumonia (LIP)
- Pneumoconiosis

Fig. 4.45 Reticulated Giraffe (photo by Dr. Folio). Note the reticulated pattern that is very similar to the reticulated septal lines on CT

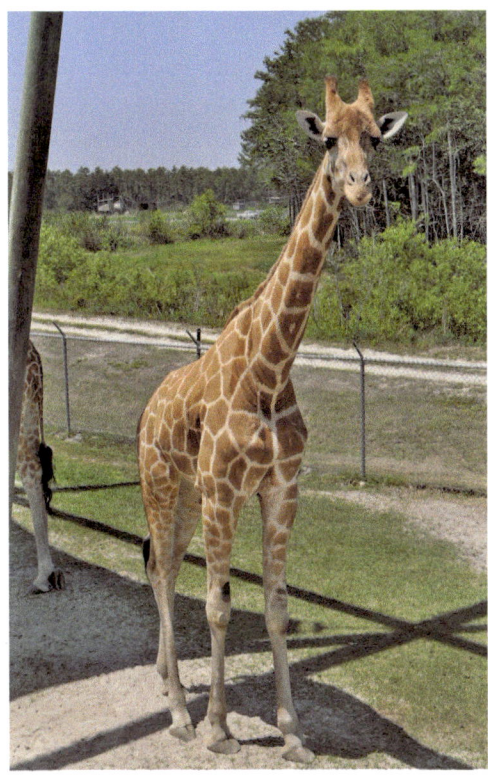

Note: One should consider the differential for mass when categorizing nodules, since they are essentially small masses.

Case 4.15

Figure 4.49 is an example of multiple, diffusely distributed nodules. Note the white dots are even in size, even when going from hila to periphery, ruling out vessels on end. This case represents Miliary Tuberculosis (TB).

Findings: Multiple, diffusely distributed nodules.

Pattern: Interstitial, specifically dots.

Differential Diagnosis: Miliary TB, histoplasmosis, coccidiomycosis, silicosis.

The miliary nodular interstitial pattern has an extensive differential; however, you can use TEMPS as a mnemonic to help you remember these causes of miliary interstitial pulmonary nodules [6].

T – TB, fungal, viral pneumonias, tuberous sclerosis

E – Eosinophilic granuloma (EG); see langerhans cell histiocytosis (LCH)

M – Metastatic disease (thyroid, renal)

P – Pneumoconioses, parasites

S – Sarcoidosis, Silicosis

Fig. 4.46 (**a**) Close-up of the giraffe; then grayscale manipulation (**b**) to increase the contrast to better simulate septal lines seen on CT (**c**) ((**a**, **b**) created by USUHS ETI Support Office)

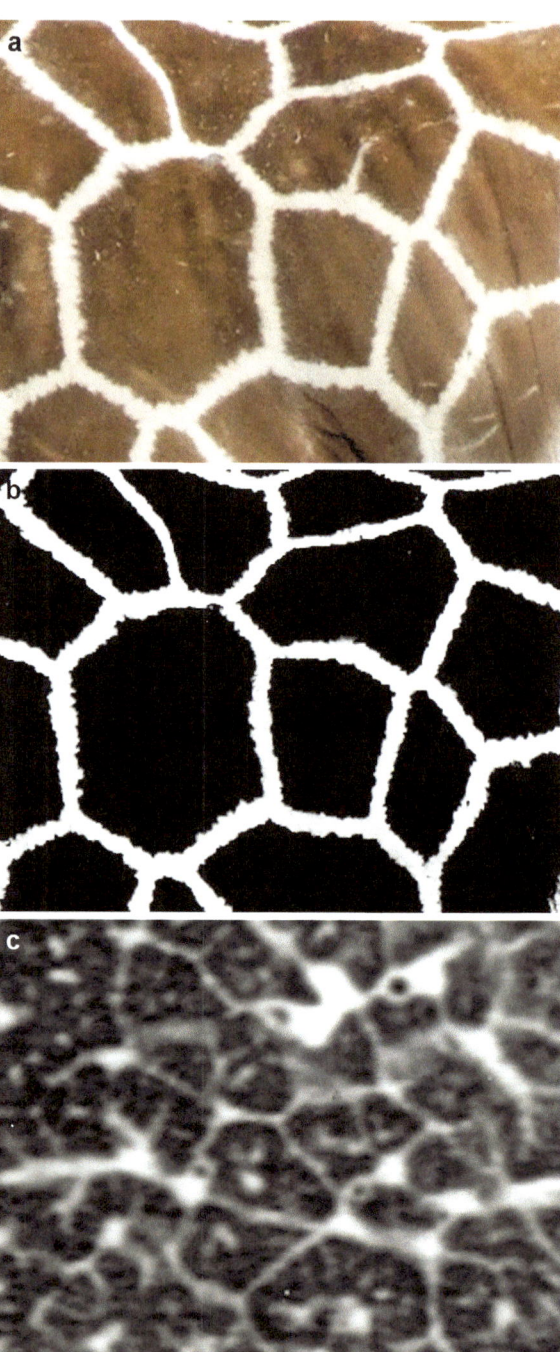

Fig. 4.47 Kerley lines (left costophrenic angle in **a**) on a dual energy (note that the ribs are digitally subtracted) CXR. Also note spine sign on lateral (**b**) supporting a right pleural effusion with atelectasis

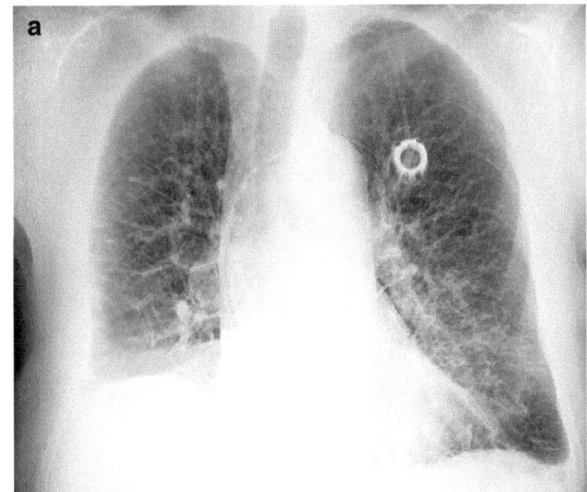

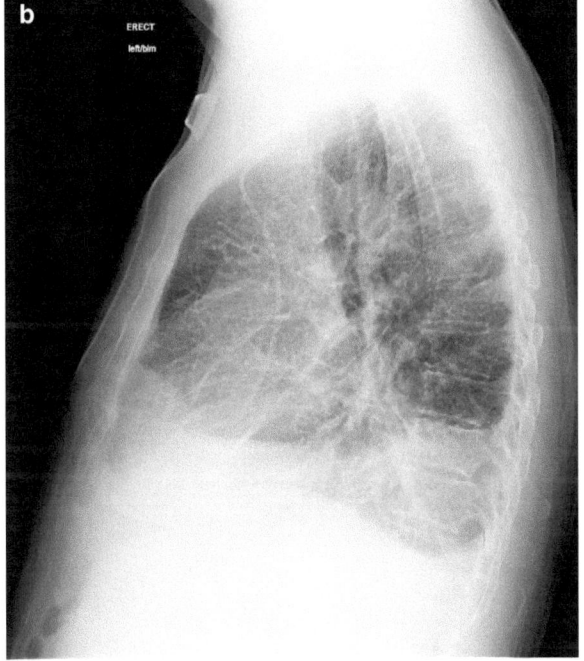

Fig. 4.48 Close-up of CXR
with Kerley lines (*arrows*)

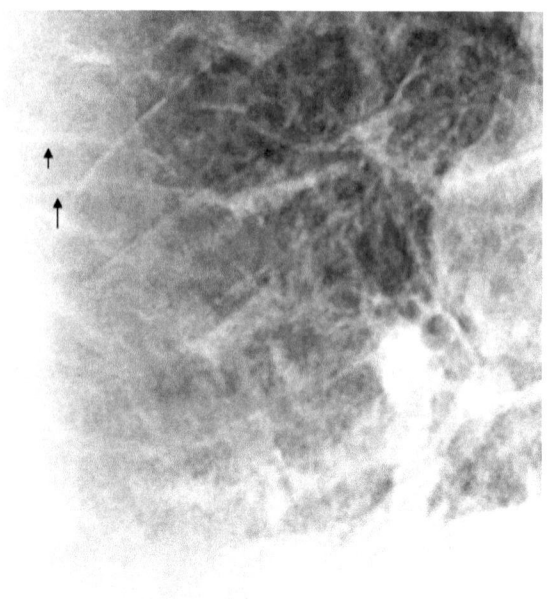

Fig. 4.49 Diffuse nodular
pattern of miliary TB

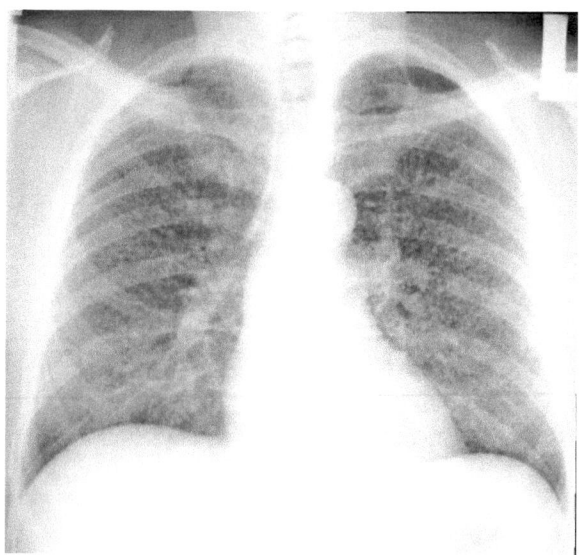

Reticulo-Nodular Form

This subcategory of interstitial markings is simply a combination of lines and dots
and has its own narrowed differential that can be remembered using the mnemonic
"PINES."[12]

P – Pneumoconiosis
I – Inflammation infection
N – Neoplasm
E – Edema
S – Sarcoidosis

Pneumoconiosis

Pneumoconiosis represents occupational lung disease caused by the inhalation of various types of industrial dust. Depending on the type of dust, variants of the disease are considered. Many cases have findings that are a combination of reticulations and nodules (reticulo-nodular).

The following mnemonic can be helpful in recalling the types of pneumoconiosis: B-CHAOS.[12]

B – Berylliosis or "benign"
C – Coal worker's pneumonoconisosis (also known as "black lung")
H – Hard metal disease
A – Asbestosis (clinical, exposure, plaques, bodies)
O – Others: Siderosis (deposition of iron in tissue), talcosis, carbon, aluminosis, kaolin
S – Silicosis (from silica dust), stannosis

Case 4.16

Figures 4.50 – 4.52 show bilateral nodules, predominantly in the upper lobes, in a patient diagnosed with coal worker's disease.

Findings: Multiple dots and lines distributed throughout the lung fields, with a coalesced opacity in the right upper lung field.

Pattern: Interstitial, specifically reticulo-nodular. One can consider the mass differential as well.

Differential Diagnosis: Coal worker's pneumoconiosis with progressive massive fibrosis (definition, when there is evidence of coalescence of nodules >1 cm). Also consider the PINES mnemonic differential.

Inflammation Infection

Case 4.17

Figures 4.53 and 4.54 is of a 60-year-old HIV-positive male with a CD4 count of 144 cells/mm^3 who was complaining of cough, dyspnea, and chest pain [2].

Fig. 4.50 CXR of coal
worker's disease (CWP)

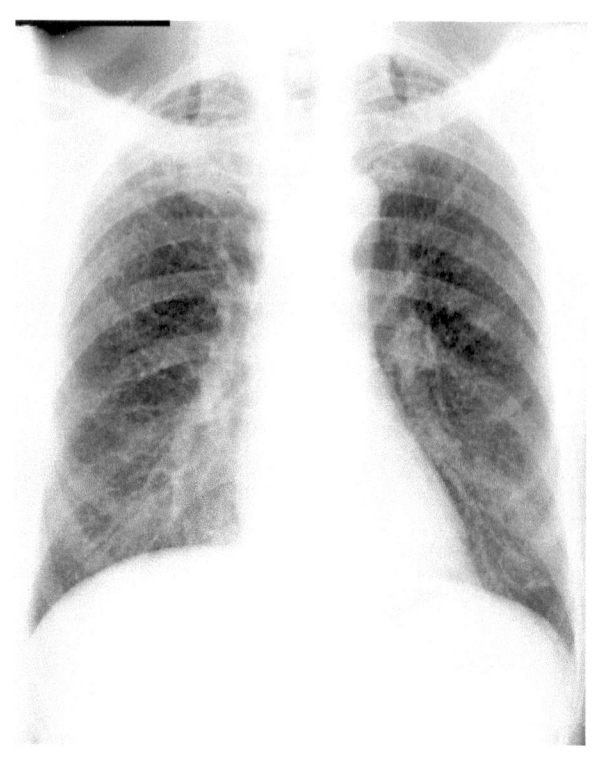

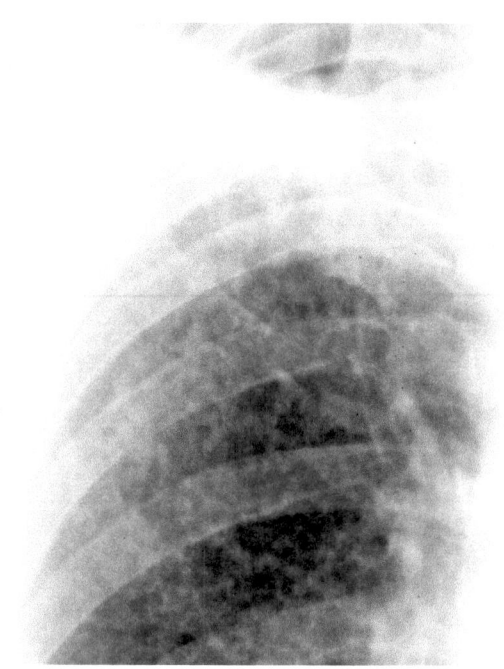

Fig. 4.51 Close-up of same
patient

Fig. 4.52 Same close-up, with nodules *circled*

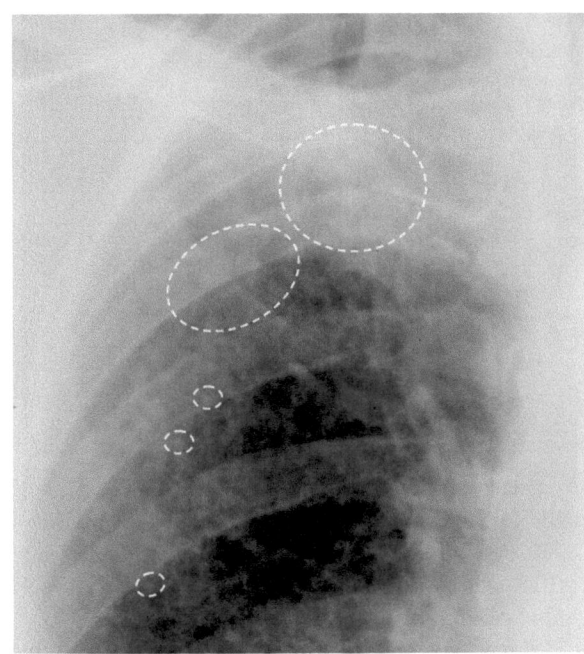

Fig. 4.53 CXR showing reticulo-nodular pattern in a patient with *Pneumocystis jiroveci* Pneumonia (PJP)

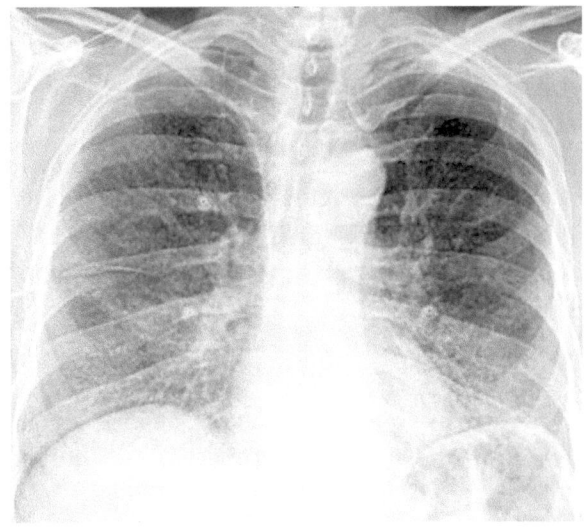

Findings: CXR and CT showing bibasilar reticulo-nodular ground-glass opacities. On CT, ground-glass attenuation and interstitial thickening in a predominantly lower lobe and dependent distribution.

  Pattern: Reticulo-nodular.

  Differential Diagnosis: *Pneumocystis jiroveci* Pneumonia (PJP).

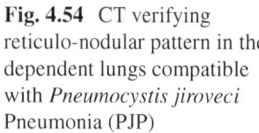

Fig. 4.54 CT verifying reticulo-nodular pattern in the dependent lungs compatible with *Pneumocystis jiroveci* Pneumonia (PJP)

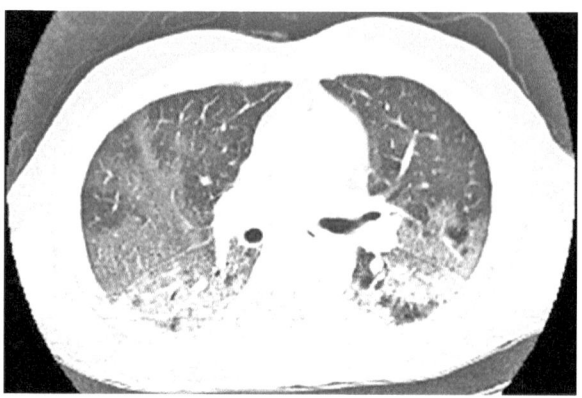

Other causes of ground-glass opacities and interstitial infiltrates in patients with AIDS include CMV pneumonia, lymphocytic interstitial pneumonia, MAI infection, cryptococcal infection, Legionella, Mycoplasma, Chlamydia pneumoniae, AIDS-related lymphoma, Kaposi sarcoma, hypersensitivity pneumonia, and interstitial pulmonary edema from volume overload.

This patient was ultimately diagnosed with PJP by lung biopsy after a negative bronchoalveolar lavage [7].

Destructive Fibrotic Lung

The destructive process of pulmonary fibrosis (lung scarring resulting in restrictive lung) progresses by scar tissue gradually replacing normal lung tissue. This eventually results in lung tissue interspersed with pockets of air (holes). This process can lead to parts of the lung having a honeycomb-like appearance, as in the next case.

Case 4.18

Figures 4.55–4.57 illustrate a case of fibrosing alveolitis and provide another example of a CXR with findings consistent with destructive findings (holes). This is most pronounced in the left lower lung.

Findings: honeycomb appearance.

Pattern: Interstitial, specifically, lines and holes.

Differential Diagnosis: Destructive lung, end-stage lung, lung fibrosis, scleroderma, LCH, LAM.

The following image is a CT of the lungs in a patient with a destructive pattern showing diffuse, stacked, irregular cyst formation.

Fig. 4.55 Fibrosing alveolitis

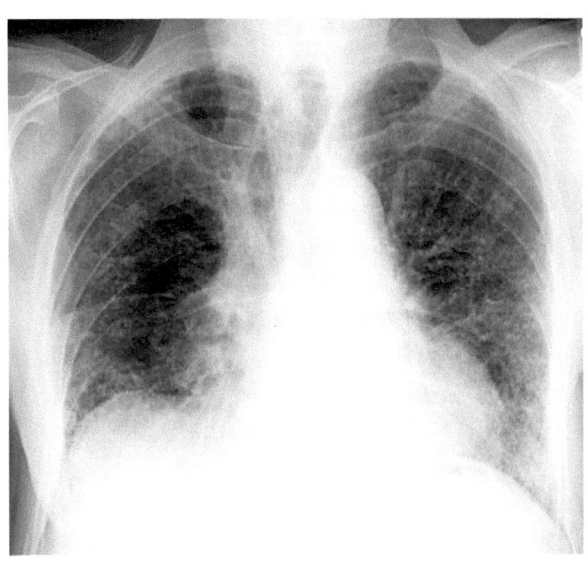

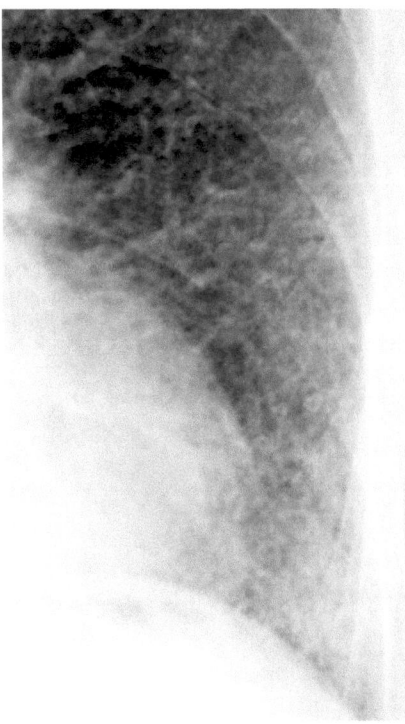

Fig. 4.56 Close-up of same patient with
fibrosing alveolitis; note the suggestion of holes
peripherally

Fig. 4.57 CT of destructive
cyst formation, honeycomb
pattern in periphery

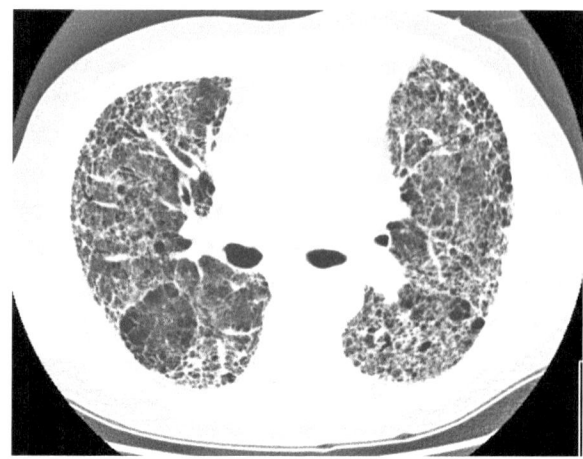

Langerhans Cell Histiocytosis

When you see lines, dots, and holes together as in the images below, think about Langerhans cell histiocytosis (LCH). One can consider the differential for each set of lines, dots, and holes; however, this would be an extensive differential diagnosis. Considerations can be narrowed based on the severity of findings, the mixture of each entity, and the clinical history.

Case 4.19

Figures 4.58 and 4.59 are from a case of LCH.
  Findings: Lines and dots diffusely distributed, with holes between lines.
  Pattern: Interstitial, specifically lines, dots, and holes.
  Differential Diagnosis: Langerhans cell histiocytosis (LCH) and LAM (lymphangi-oleiomyomatosis). Again, one could consider an exhaustive differential (all of intersti-tial); however, the combination of lines, dots, and holes is typically seen in LCH.
  Open lung biopsy supported LCH.

Vascular Pattern

Normal Pulmonary Vascular Anatomic Review

As mentioned previously, normal pulmonary markings (vessels, arteries for the most part) can typically be followed from the hilum toward the lung periphery in all directions. They branch at acute angles, taper, and diverge toward the periphery.

Fig. 4.58 CXR showing *lines*, *dots*, and *holes* together

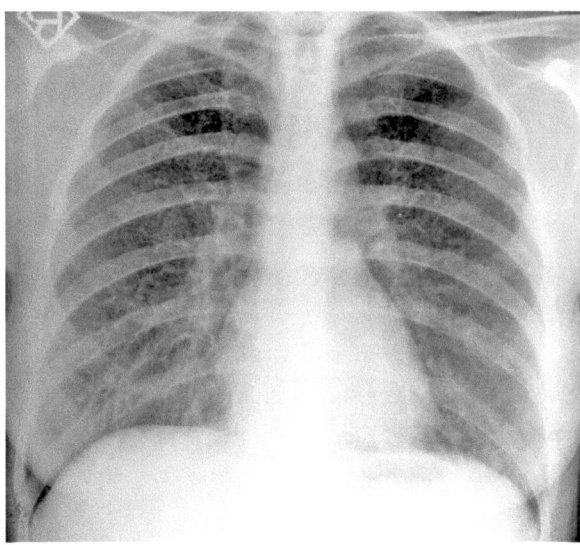

Fig. 4.59 Close-up of CXR showing lines, dots, and holes

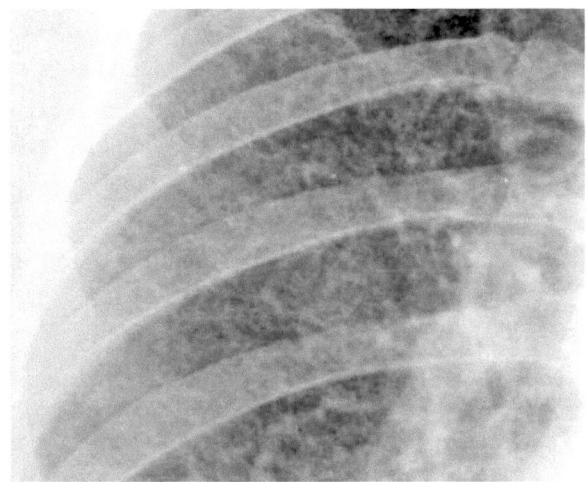

Pulmonary markings on-end appear as small masses or nodules. They are recognized as normal vessels by the fact that they are often superimposed upon vessels of the same diameter branching in other directions. They are also larger toward the hilum and similarly sized to vessels nearby.

Radiological Signs in the Vascular Pattern

Abnormal diameter or distribution/ distortion of pulmonary vasculature.

Mechanism

Vascular process can be evident with increased or decreased perfusion, and/ or altering diameter of pulmonary vessels. Additionally, distortion from masses or bullae is possible.

In review, the vascular pattern includes processes that effect the visualization of vasculature, however, may not be primarily vascular etiology.

Vascular Examples

There are a number of conditions altering vasculature, hence qualifying for the vascular pattern. Three conditions affecting the CXR are presented, including:

1. *Pulmonary Arterial Hypertension*: Large central arteries with peripheral tapering
2. *Congestion*: Engorged veins, especially upper lungs
3. *Emphysema*: Diminished or compresses or distorted vasculature

   Other conditions include:

- *Lymphangitic Carcinoma*: Irregular infiltration around vessels may resemble vessel enlargement.
- *Thromboembolism*: Locally diminished vessels with possible vessel mass centrally located.
- *Bronchial Circulation*: Irregular vessels in unusual directions.
- *Shunt Vascularity*: All vessels enlarged.

Pulmonary Arterial Hypertension (PAH)

PAH presents large central arteries with peripheral tapering. Think about conditions such as chronic thrombophlebitis and, secondarily, obesity (Pickwickianism) and sleep apnea.

Pulmonary arterial hypertension (PAH) is continuous high blood pressure in the pulmonary artery. The average blood pressure in a normal pulmonary artery is about 15 mmHg when the person is resting. In PAH, the average is usually greater than 25 mmHg [8].

In PAH, three types of changes may occur in the pulmonary arteries.

1. The muscles within the walls of the arteries may tighten up. This makes the inside of the arteries narrower.
2. The walls of the pulmonary arteries may thicken as the amount of muscle increases in some arteries. Scar tissue may form in the walls of arteries. As the walls thicken and scar, the arteries become increasingly narrow.
3. Tiny blood clots may form within the smaller arteries, causing blockages [8].

Case 4.20

Figure 4.60 illustrates PAH with tapering vessels (often referred to as "pruning") using an analogy with a tree that was pruned.

The tree in Fig. 4.60b was pruned and now has small branches growing from the stumps, not dissimilar to how enlarged pulmonary arteries abruptly taper with small branches emanating after the elasticity changes to the intima.

Figures 4.61a and 4.62a demonstrate an enlarged pulmonary trunk, sometimes known as a middle mogul.

Findings: Enlarged pulmonary arteries proximally with tapering peripherally.
Pattern: Vascular.
Differential Diagnosis: PAH, COPD, cor pulmonale.

Fig. 4.60a This CXR shows enlarged pulmonary arteries bilaterally. Note how quickly the arteries taper to thinner branches

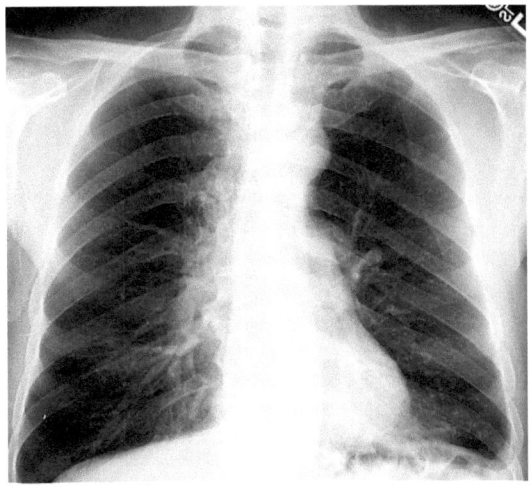

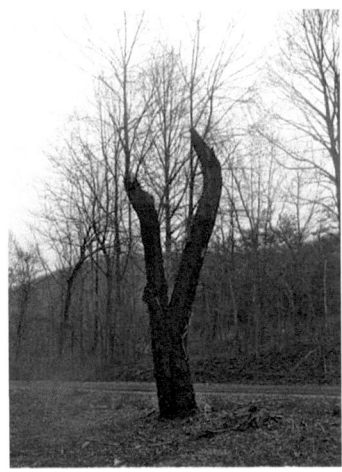

Fig. 4.60b This photo of a pruned tree shows some smaller branches that have grown since the pruning (Photos by Dr. Les Folio)

Fig. 4.60c Same photo, only reversed in black and white to create the following collage

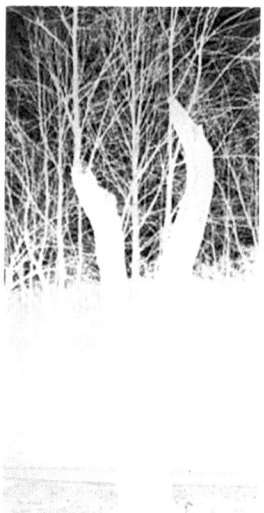

Fig. 4.60d The CXR of PAH with manipulated pruned trees to demonstrate pruning model

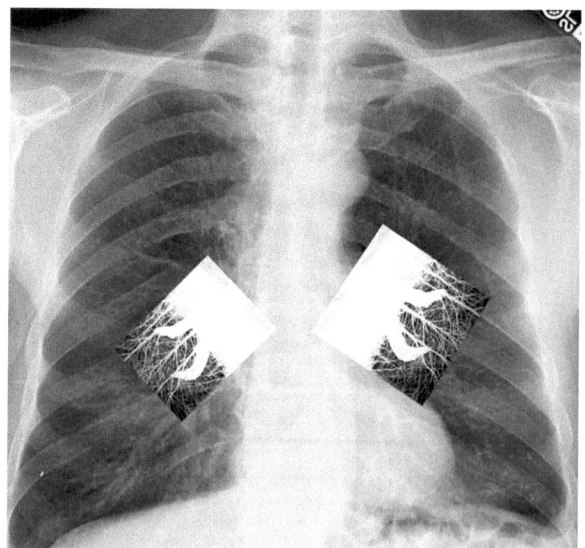

"Hypoxic vasoconstriction, obliteration of the pulmonary vascular bed, and volume overload are the three core pathophysiologic processes that lead to pulmonary artery hypertension."

"Hypoxic vasoconstriction occurs most commonly in the setting of chronic obstructive pulmonary disease. Chronic hypoxia leads to vasoconstriction of the pulmonary vasculature, which leads to pulmonary artery hypertension. Similarly, if there is a 60% or greater loss of the total pulmonary vasculature (obliteration of the pulmonary vascular bed), pulmonary artery hypertension will ensue. This is common in patients with chronic pulmonary emboli and collagen vascular disorders."

"A multitude of cardiac disorders can lead to elevated pulmonary arterial pressures. Several stem from disorders affecting the left heart. Mitral and aortic valvular disease along with cardiomyopathies increase the pulmonary pressure gradient over time and lead to pulmonary artery hypertension. Pulmonary volume overload occurs with congenital heart diseases such as Atrial Septal Defect (ASD) or Ventricular Septal Defect (VSD) causing left to right shunts [9]."

Figure 4.62c is a 37-year-old female (different patient from above) with large MPA on CXR, suspected of having a pulmonary embolus.

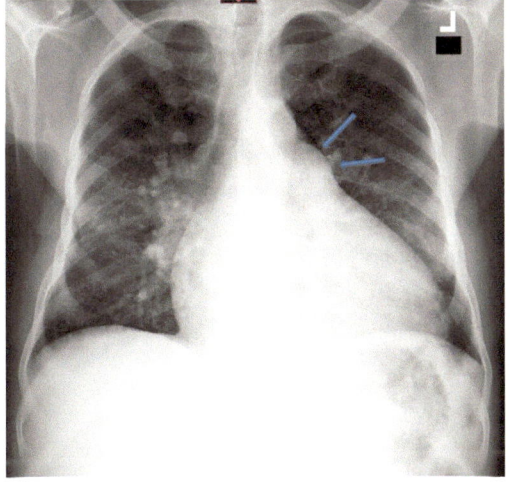

Fig. 4.61a PA of a 34-year-old male patient with sickle cell anemia and PAH. Note the large main pulmonary trunk (*arrows*). The cardiac silhouette is also enlarged

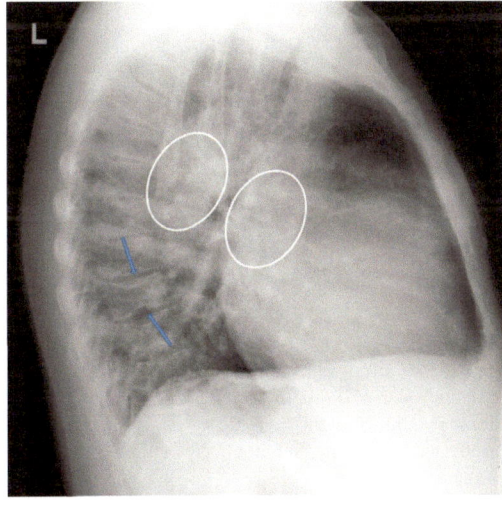

Fig. 4.61b Lateral of same patient showing large left (*posterior circle*) and right (*anterior circle*) pulmonary arteries. Also note the typical H-shaped vertebral bodies of sickle cell disease

Fig. 4.61c HRCT (*done prone*)
demonstrating mosaic attenuation
(*previously known as mosaic
"perfusion" or mosaicism*). The *two
arrows* contrast the whiter versus
darker lung in this pattern often seen
with PAH due to perfusion variation.
Also note the large segmental and
subsegmental pulmonary arteries

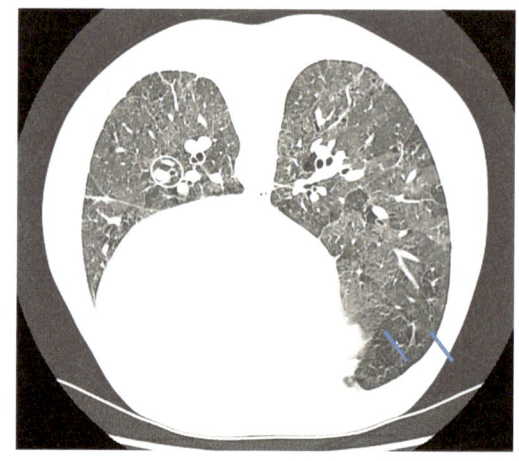

Fig. 4.62a Enlarged
pulmonary trunk on axial CT
thick slab MIP (Maximum
Intensity Projection) in a
patient with lung metastasis.
Note the larger Main
Pulmonary Artery (trunk, or
MPA) over the Aorta (*A*).
Note the masses (*M*) and
effusions (*eff*)

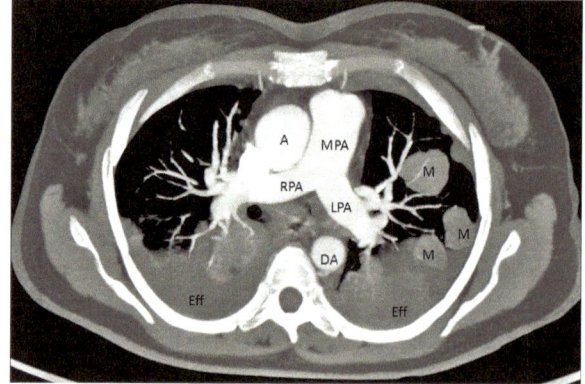

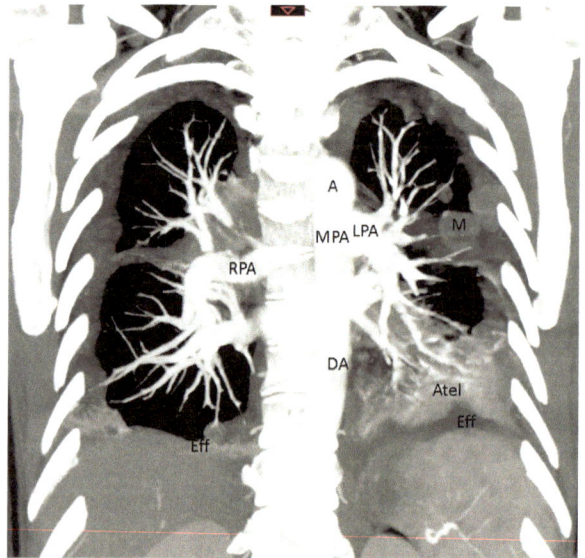

Fig. 4.62b Enlarged
pulmonary arteries on coronal
CT thick slab MIP in the
same patient. Note the
truncated branching. Note the
atelectasis (*atel*) LLL
adjacent to the effusion (*eff*)

Fig. 4.62c PA CXR
demonstrating large MPA
mogul (*large arrows*) and
large right interlobar
pulmonary artery (*small
arrows*).

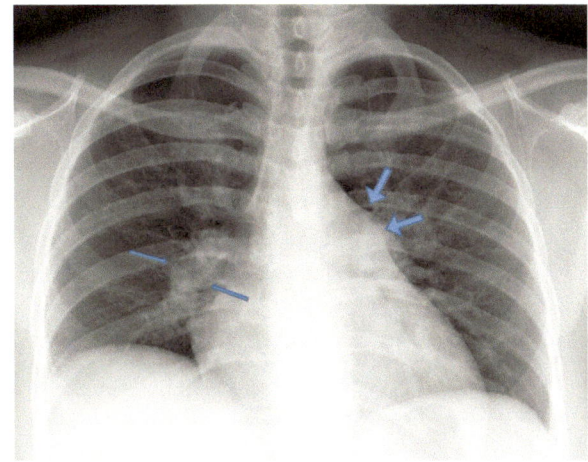

Fig. 4.62d Axial CT
reformatted 20 mm slab of
same patient showing a wall
adherent thrombus (*arrows*)
of the right interlobar
pulmonary artery (*RILPA*).
Also note the large left lower
lobe pulmonary artery
(*LLLPA*) and corkscrew
peripheral pulmonary arteries
(*dotted circle*) in LLL. Also
noted is the right atrium (*RA*),
right ventricle (*RV*), left
atrium (*LA*), left ventricle
(*LV*), right main pulmonary
artery (*RPA*), and left
pulmonary vein (*LPV*)

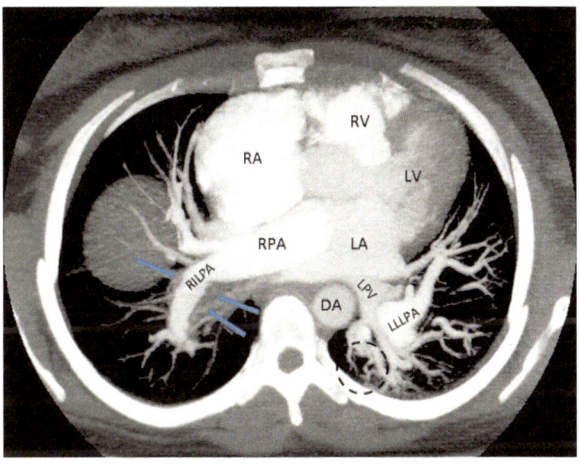

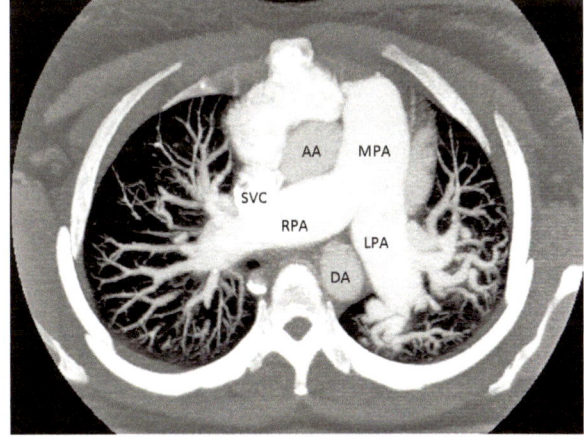

Fig. 4.62e Axial CT
reformatted 20 mm slab at
level of enlarged MPA and
enlarged central pulmonary
arteries (*RPA, LPA*). Also
note large pulmonary artery
braches bilaterally, and
corkscrewing again on the
left. Ascending aorta (*AA*)
and descending aorta and
superior vena cava (*SVC*) also
seen

Fig. 4.62f Coronal CT
showing large pulmonary
artery (2.9 cm) relative to
aorta (2.4 cm) and mosaic
attenuation of lungs
bilaterally

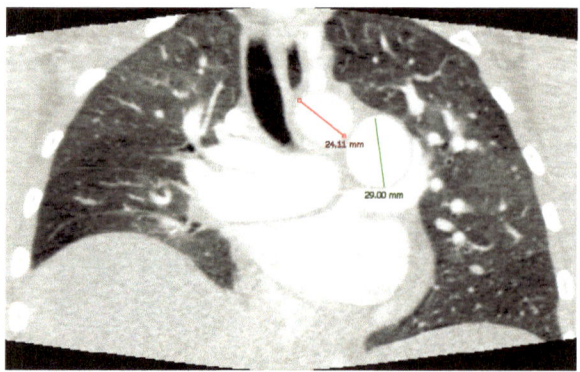

Fig. 4.63 Congested
vasculature in this patient
with edema

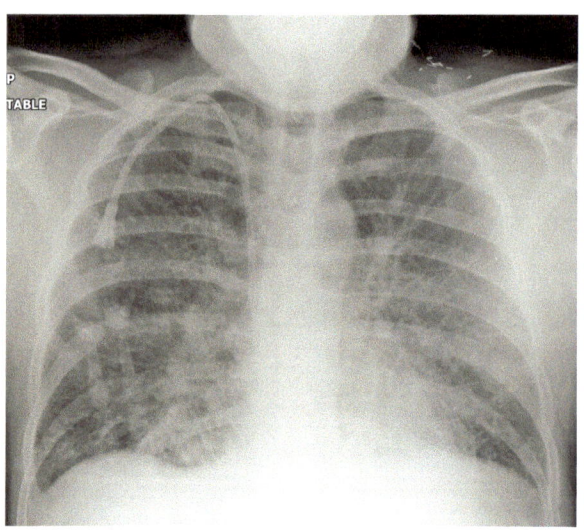

Pulmonary Venous Congestion

Variations in pulmonary blood flow (arteries or veins) can help narrow differential
diagnosis to pulmonary and cardiac processes. For example, vascular congestion in
the form of pulmonary venous congestion can help track the prognosis on ICU
patients with primary vascular/cardiac issues versus overflow issues from other
processes.

Figure 4.63 depicts a congested vasculature pattern. Notice the engorged veins,
especially in the upper lungs.

Findings: Increased pulmonary vasculature.

Pattern: Vascular.

Differential Diagnosis: PVH, CHF, ARDS.

Fig. 4.64 Interstitial edema, note the fine interstitial markings in increasing opacifying lungs. Note adequately placed ET and NG tubes. Right IJ line in SVC (rotated projection)

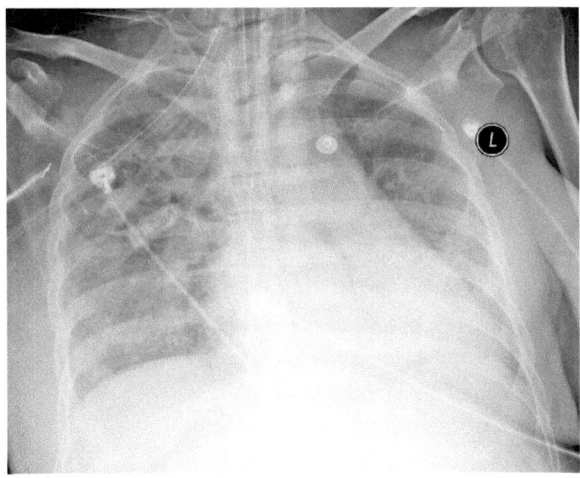

Pulmonary Venous Congestion: Edema

Figure 4.64 depicts a diffuse, fine reticular pattern with a differential diagnosis of exudates, transudate, hemorrhage, secretions, or malignancy. Although not a vascular pattern, the interstitial pattern is compatible with ARDS.

Emphysema

Although not primarily a vascular condition, emphysema can cause extrinsic pressure to vasculature, causing a compressed and distorted appearance to the pulmonary vasculature in the apicies leading to this diagnosis.

Figure 4.65a provides an example of compressed vessels; decreased diameter of vessels is caused by excessive air pressure around them.

Findings: Upper lobe diminished and distorted vessels.

Pattern: Vascular.

Differential Diagnosis: Bullous emphysema, COPD.

Airway (Bronchial) Patterns

For a brief description and graphic of normal airways, see the normal lung markings page of this book.

Mechanisms
- Complete or partial obstruction of airways
- Thickening of airway walls
- Atelectasis literally means incomplete expansion or loss of volume

Fig. 4.65a CXR showing diminished and distorted vasculature in upper lobes (*arrows*)

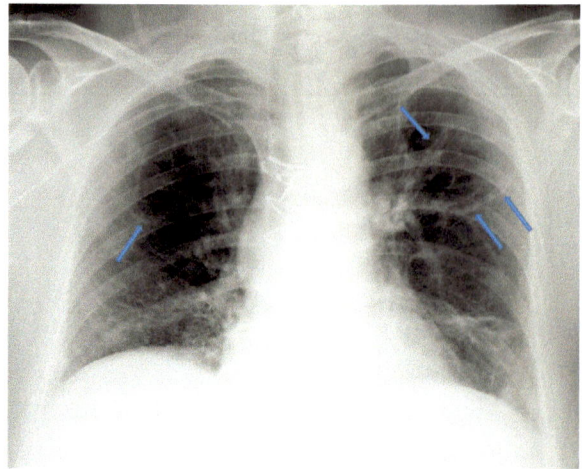

Fig. 4.65b Axial CT showing better detail of compressed and distorted vessels due to biapical bullous emphysema

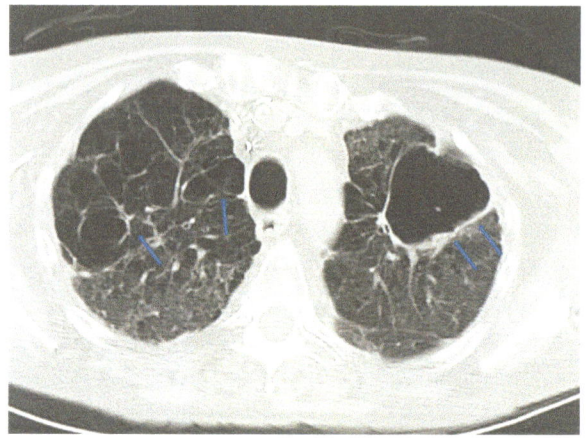

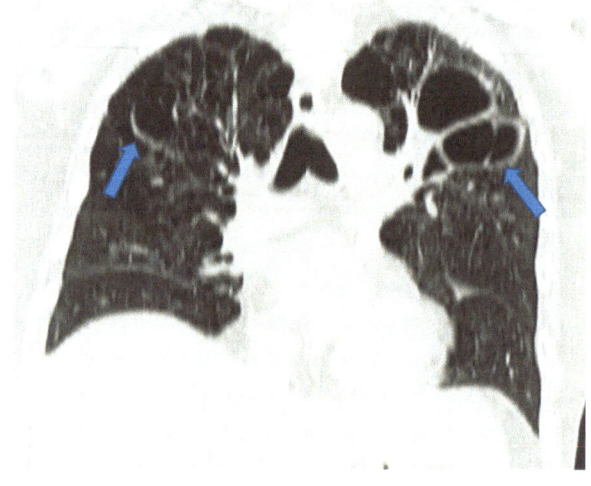

Fig. 4.65c Coronal reformat again demonstrating compressed, distorted pulmonary vasculature (*arrows*)

Forms
- Complete airway obstruction: Opacity and decreased volume
- Partial obstruction: Lucency and increased volume
- Wall thickening: Tram tracks, central cystic spaces or circles

For the differential diagnosis, look for the following.
- *Opacities*: Endobronchial malignancies; granulomas; inflammatory, benign or congenital masses; mucous plugs; foreign bodies potentially causing complete obstruction
- *Lucencies*: Chronic obstructive pulmonary disease (COPD), cysts, blebs, pneumatoceles
- *Thickening*: Bronchiectasis, chronic bronchitis

Complete Obstruction

Obstruction of a bronchus or airway results in complete obstruction.

Radiological Signs
- *Direct Signs*: Displacement of interlobar fissures
- *Indirect Signs*: Opacification, mediastinal shift (ipsilateral), hilar displacement, elevation of hemidiaphragm, crowded vasculature, compensatory hyperinflation of unaffected lung, "shifting" granuloma sign and juxtaphrenic peak

The four main types of mechanisms of obstruction and resultant atelectasis are as follows:

1. *Resorptive/Obstructive*: This type is caused by a complete bronchial obstruction. If there is no flow, then air becomes absorbed from the lung. Oxygen gets absorbed much more rapidly than ambient air. (E.g., a ventilator patient on 100% oxygen will collapse within minutes to hours.)
2. *Passive/Compressive*: This type is caused by extrinsic pressure from air, fluid, or mass (tumors, bullae, or abscesses). A large pleural fluid collection or pneumothorax could produce virtual complete collapse of the lobe.
3. *Cicatricial*: Areas of pulmonary fibrosis can cause reduced alveolar volume. It can be focal or diffuse. When focal, it is generally associated with old granulomatous infection, typically TB. However, it may be diffuse, as seen typically in idiopathic pulmonary fibrosis.
4. *Adhesive*: This type occurs in association with surfactant deficiency and subsequent microatelectasis. Type II pneumocytes can be injured from inhaled anesthetic agents, ischemia, or radiation, therefore, causes include general anesthesia, adult respiratory distress syndrome, hyaline membrane disease, and acute radiation pneumonits.

Lobar Atelectasis (Collapse)

Atelectasis literally means incomplete expansion or loss of volume.

Signs

Primary
• Vessel asymmetry
• Fissure appears as an edge

Secondary
• Volume loss
• Elevation of diaphragm
• Shift of mediastinum and ribs
    Patterns of lobar atelectasis as seen on CXRs are presented in the image below.

Lobar Atelectasis Patterns

The following figures and descriptions provide examples of the patterns of lobar atelectasis.

1. *Right Upper Lobe (RUL*, Fig. 4.66)
    Collapse is superior and medially and creates a wedge-shaped opacity in the right upper paramediastinal area on the frontal projection. The major fissure is displaced anteriorly and the minor fissure superiorly. There may be a triangular opacity with apex pointing toward hilum on lateral view. There is tracheal deviation to the right and superior displacement of the hilum. The right hemidiaphragm may be elevated. If there is a large central obstructing mass causing the atelectasis, you may have a convex bulge into the central medial portion of the displaced minor fissure. This will give a "Reverse S-sign of Golden." There may be focal diaphragmatic tenting (juxtaphrenic peak sign) which is most commonly traction on the inferior accessory fissure.

2. *Left Upper Lobe (LUL*, Fig. 4.67)
    Due to lack of a left minor fissure, the appearance of LUL collapse is much different than RUL, except when an accessory left minor fissure is present. In such a case, the upper division of the LUL atelectasis will look like RUL atelectasis. Otherwise, the left major fissure is displaced anteriorly, roughly parallel to the anterior chest wall, and there is a band of opacity anterior to the major fissure. On the PA view, there is a hazy opacity that silhouettes the left heart border.

3. and 4. *Lower Lobes (LLs*, Figs. 4.68 and 4.69)
    This pattern is similar in both the right and left lower lobes. Collapse is in posterior, medial, and inferior direction. The major fissure swings downward and backward. The hilum is displaced inferiorly, the hemidiaphragm is elevated. On the PA view,

Fig. 4.66 Example of RUL collapse

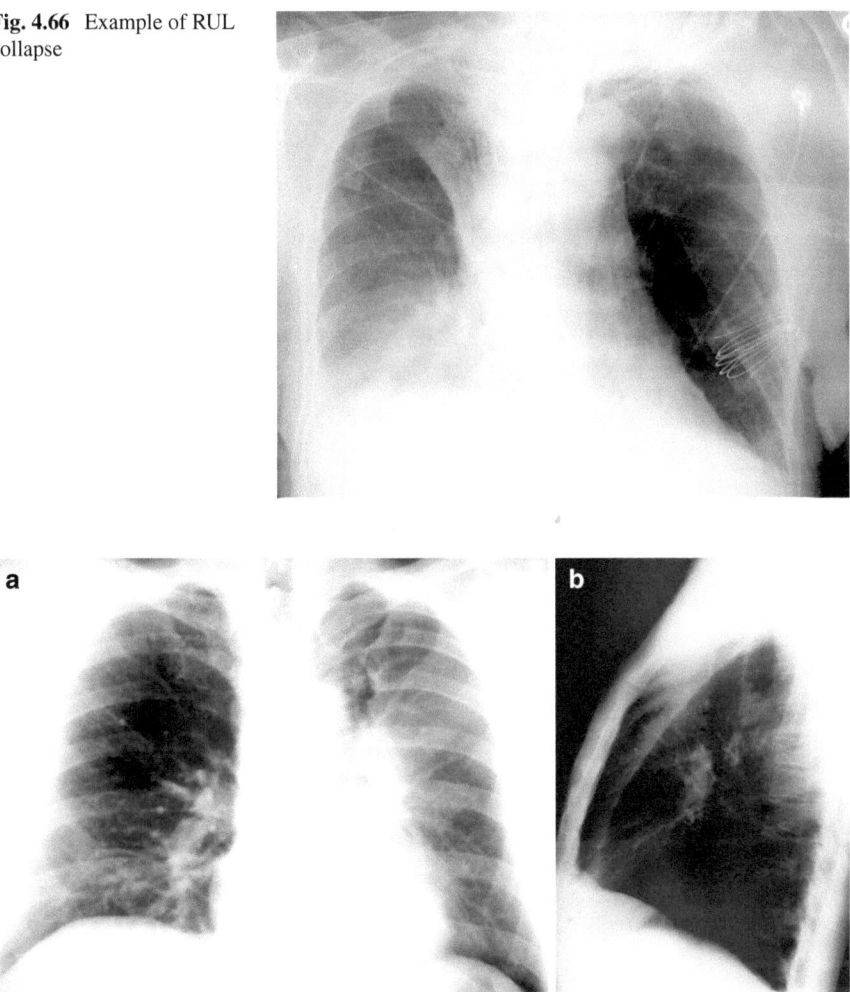

Fig. 4.67 Example of LUL collapse, AP (**a**) and lateral (**b**) projections. Note the overall increased density of the left hemithorax is due to the LUL collapsing anteriorly as seen on the lateral projection

there is a triangular opacity adjacent to the spine with the base on the hemidiaphragm. On the lateral view, there is increased opacity over the lower thoracic vertebrae with or without a smooth anterior margin, depending upon if the major fissure is tangential to the X-ray beam. The posterior aspect of the hemidiaphragm is obscured, unless the patient has an incomplete pulmonary ligament. Another indirect sign is the vascular nodular sign, which is a result of compensatory hyperinflation of the upper lobe. This is radiographically seen as "hair-pin" turning of vessels and "too-many nodules" along the cardiac margin, which are end-on vessels. Kattan's triangle sign, which is the shifted v-shaped opacity superior to the anterior junction line, may also be seen.

Fig. 4.68 Example of RLL collapse

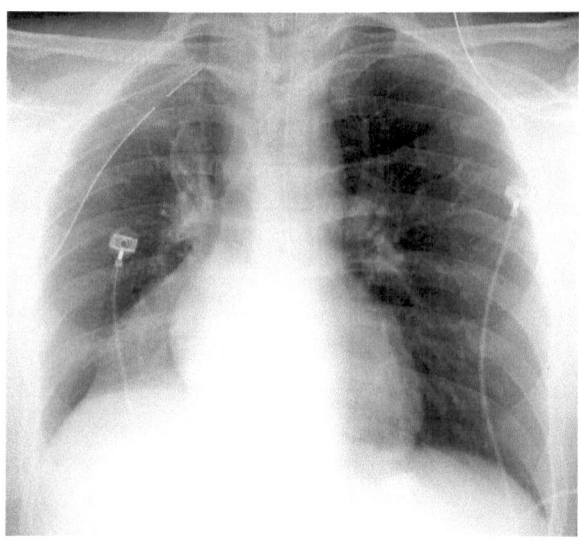

Fig. 4.69 Example of LLL collapse

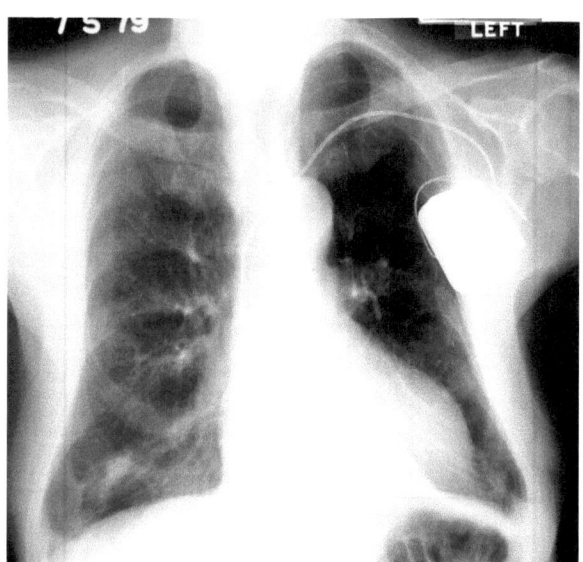

Complete Obstruction: Case Study

Figure 4.71 depicts case of developing lobar atelectasis resulting from a gunshot wound (GSW) and recovery following therapeutic bronchoscopy.

Findings: Fracture of the right mandible caused by the entry of the bullet. A bullet fragment is lodged in the trachea at the level of C2–C3. Also, notice that the arrow "RLL Atelectasis" in the first image on this page points to an ill-defined opacity of the right lower lobe. The right hemidiaphragm is elevated while the cardiac silhouette, the right atrial border in particular, is maintained. There is obvious developing opacifica-

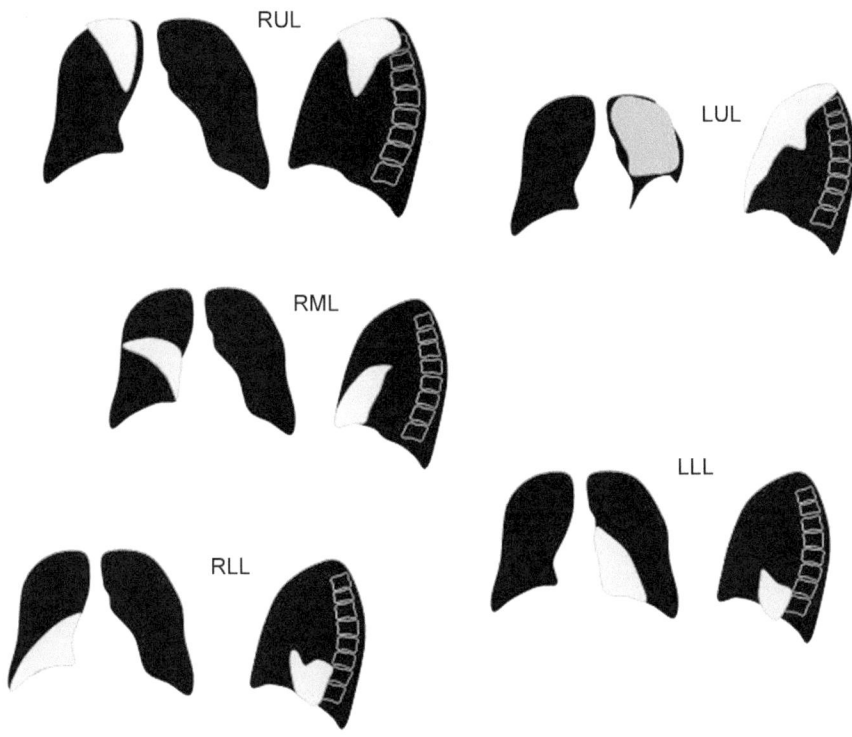

Fig. 4.70 Drawings depict the patterns of atelectasis (by Sofia Echelmeyer)

tion of the right lower lobe with obliteration of the right hemidiaphragm and the right costophrenic angle. Also, the right heart border is becoming obscured. The CXR taken several hours later displays complete collapse of the right lung.

Pattern: Airway, complete obstruction.

Differential Diagnosis: RLL atelectasis from obstruction from blood, bullet fragments, or tooth (blood most likely since metal or calcification is not seen in the area of the bronchus). A blood clot was discovered and removed at urgent bronchoscopy.

Aspiration, potentially developing into pneumonia; however, post bronchoscopy CXR shows clearing after removal of blood.

Partial Obstruction

A good example of partial airway obstruction is bronchiolitis obliterans (BO) where air-trapping can be seen on expiration CT. This condition is uncommon; however, this can be seen post infection, especially in children, or post transplant. See Fig. 4.72 for inspiration/expiration HRCT demonstrating air-trapping in the expiration.

Fig. 4.71a CT scout of head, neck, and chest showing a GSW to the mandible with the bullet in the trachea. Note developing RLL atelectasis

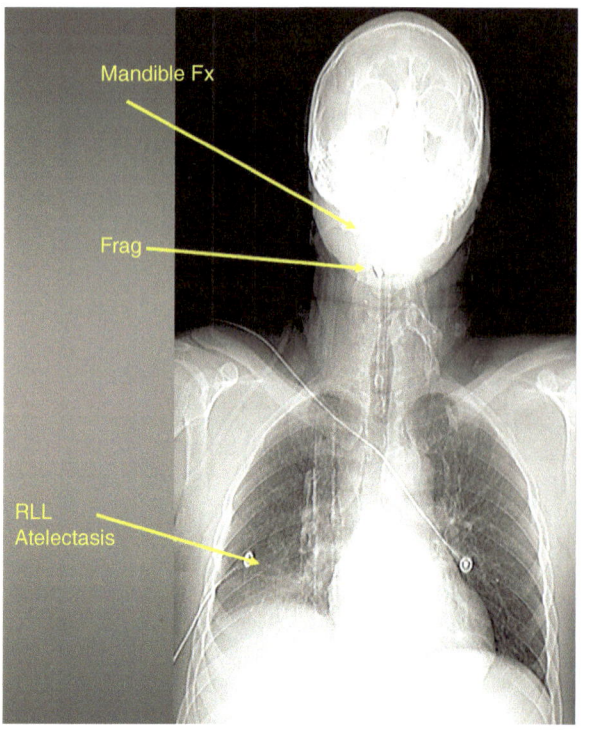

Fig. 4.71b CXR obtained 1 h after GSW showing decreased visualization of the right hemidiaphragm with associated increasing density RLL

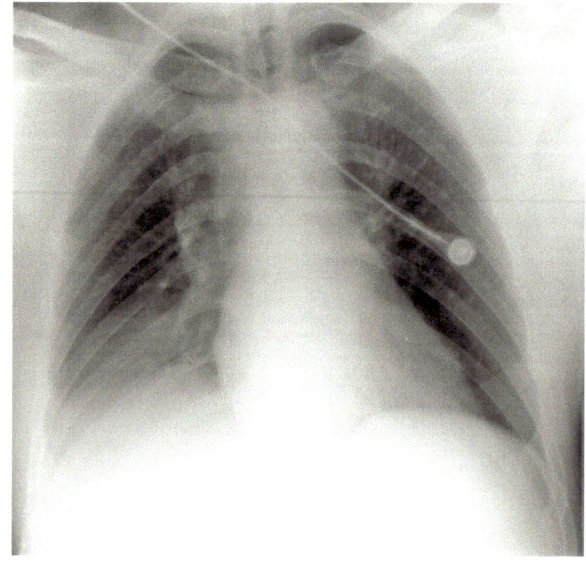

Fig. 4.71c CXR obtained in ICU 3 h after wound showing complete whiteout of right hemithorax with truncation of right mainstem bronchus. Note also shift in the trachea to the right. This is compatible with right lung collapse due to right mainstem bronchus obstruction

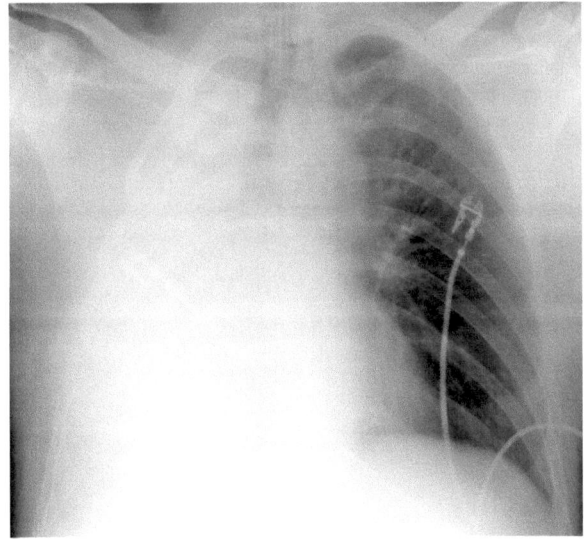

Fig. 4.71d CXR post bronchoscopy/removal of blood clot. Note the return of aeration to the right lung

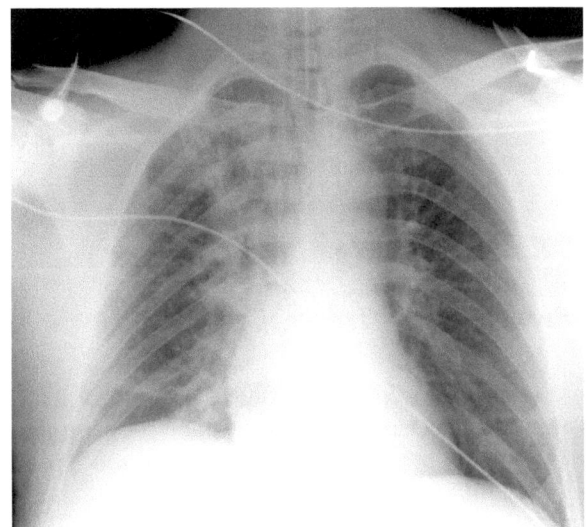

Radiological Signs

Can also have increased lung volume (chronic air-trapping) overall.
   Findings: Generalized hyperaeration, with additional localized air collections.
   Pattern: Airway, partial obstruction.

Differential Diagnosis
- Bronchiolitis obliterans
- COPD
- Centrilobular emphysema
- Pneumatoceles

Fig. 4.72 Inspiration (**a**) and
expiration (**b**) HRCT
demonstrating lucency from
air-trapping on the expiration
CT (*arrows* in **b**) due to
bronchiolitis obliterans

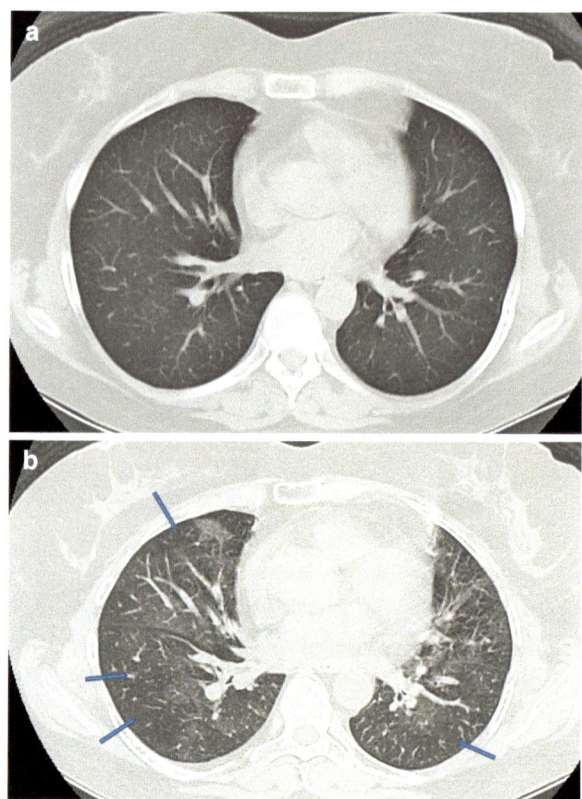

Bronchial Wall Thickening

The following section starts with causes of bronchial wall thickening, findings, and
an analog to demonstrate why the findings appear the way they do.

Bronchial Wall Thickening Causes

Bronchial wall thickening (bronchiectasis) involves a large differential diagnosis.
Table 4.2 contains a complete list of causes.

Figure 4.73 is an example case from a patient with cystic fibrosis.

Bronchial Wall Thickening Model

Figures 4.74 and 4.75a are presented as a model to help explain bronchial wall
thickening. This was published by Slotto and Folio and reprinted with permission [5].

Table 4.2 Causes of bronchiectasis

Congenital	Cystic fibrosis
	Kartagener's syndrome
	Alpha-1-antitrypsin deficiency
	Bronchomalacia
	Yellow nail syndrome
Severe inflammation	Mycobacterium (i.e., tuberculosis) or NTM (Non-TB mycobacterium)
	MRSA
	Toxoplasmosis, rubella, CMV, herpes simplex, syphilis (TORCHES)
	Fungal infection
Obstructive	Foreign body aspiration
	Bronchial stricture
	Airway mass/tumor
	External compression

Reprinted with permission from Slotto and Folio [5]
For organizational purposes, it is useful to divide bronchial wall thickening into the three broad categories shown on the *left*. Within each category, the most common disease entities are shown on the *right*

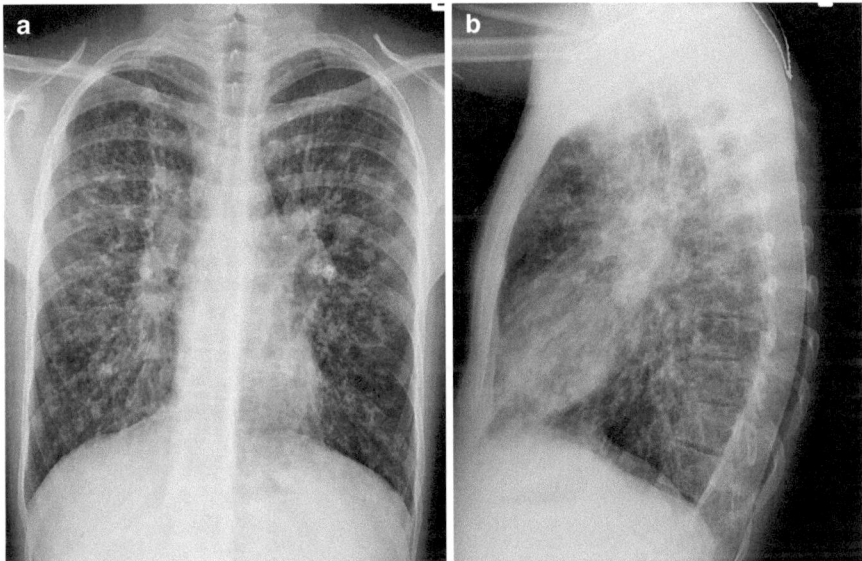

Fig. 4.73 Note the diffuse tram tracks and *peribronchial cuffing* representing the thickened bronchial walls on PA (**a**) and lateral (**b**). See the following analog for more detail of the findings

Figure 4.74 are gross photos of the experimental setup for plain computed radiography. The green sponge has contrast medium on half, and the blue has been soaked with water to better simulate tissue density.

Figure 4.75a shows the tram track in the experimental model, with plain film to the left and axial CT on the right. The plain film shows one straw in profile (left) and

Fig. 4.74 Experimental setup for bronchial wall thickening model. Plain computed radiography (*CR*, **a**) and CT (**b**) were obtained of a sponge and an apple with straws piercing through to demonstrate air bronchograms (*apple*) and tram tracks (*sponge*) by analogy

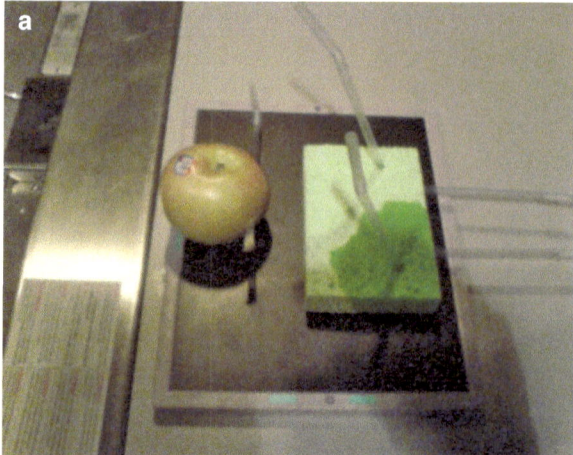

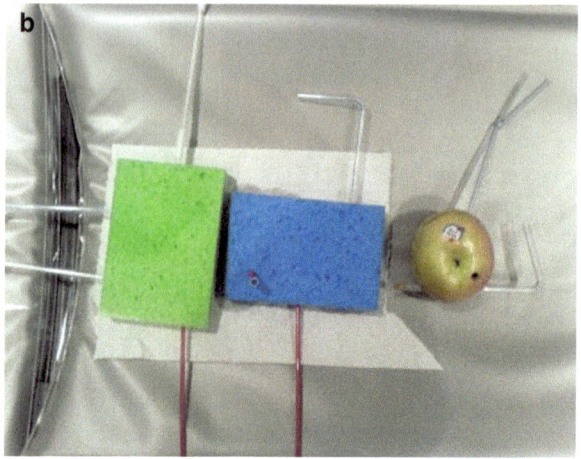

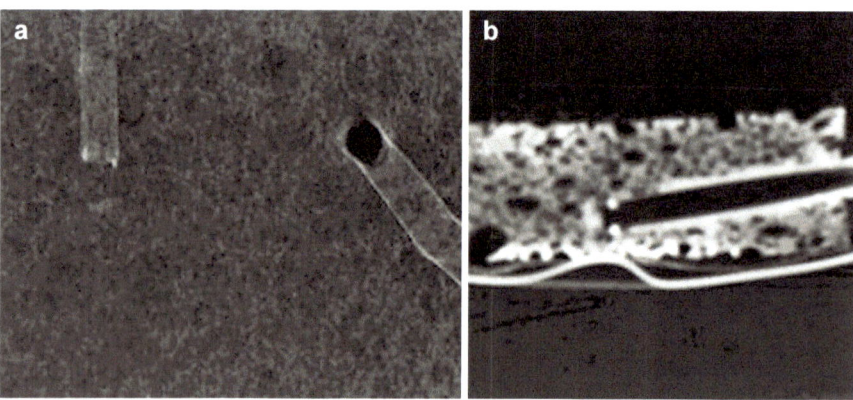

Fig. 4.75a, b Tram track in experimental model. The plain CR image (**a**) is not as revealing as the CT (**b**)

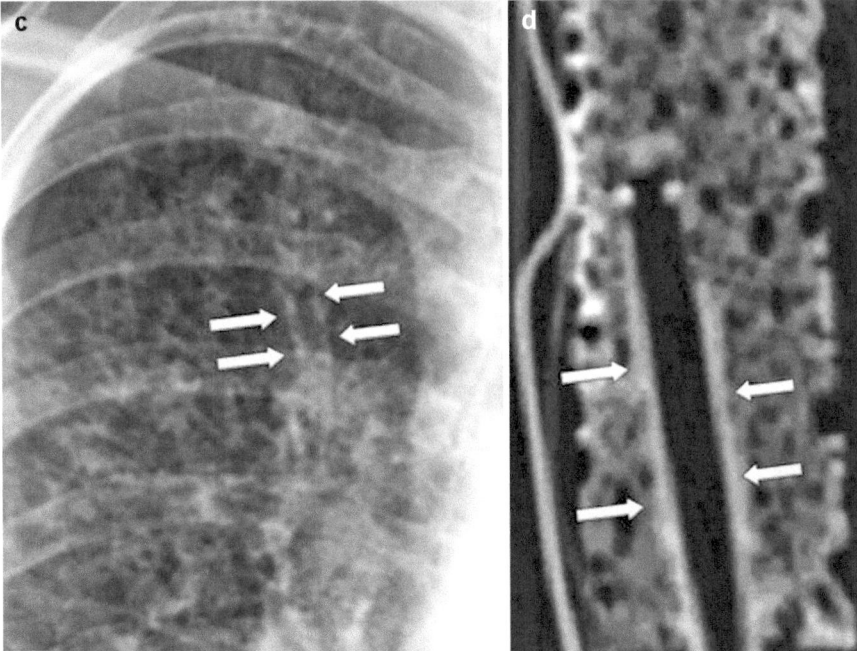

Fig. 4.75c, d Tram tracks in our patient (*left image*, **c**) and experimental analog with straw and sponge (*right image*, **d**)

one straw in oblique (right). The CT image shows the increased attenuation of the tape-wrapped straw mimicking bronchial wall thickening.

Side-by-side comparison of the in vivo tram track sign on the left and the experimental analog on the right. The arrows point to the thickened bronchiole walls seen in the CF patient, created in the same fashion by a straw wrapped in tape producing a thick wall around a hollow tube inside the sponge.

Figure 4.76a shows a CT of the chest in a patient with bronchiectasis, with obvious signet ring signs indicating bronchial dilation relative to the pulmonary arteries.

Figure 4.76b, c show the experimental model image using the sponge. There are two parallel straws of different diameters, the smaller having been filled with radio-opaque material to simulate adjacent vessel, the large straw with air to represent enlarged bronchiole.

Bronchiolar

Radiological signs of a small airway obstruction are airway ("alveolar") nodules, irregular in size, shape, and distribution; and, small, irregular lucencies. You can see a "Tree-in-bud" appearance on CT. This looks like branches of trees in the spring that start budding, typically only seen on CT.

Fig. 4.76a CT of bronchial
dilation (bronchus is larger
than the companion artery).
Note the tracheomalacia of
the carina

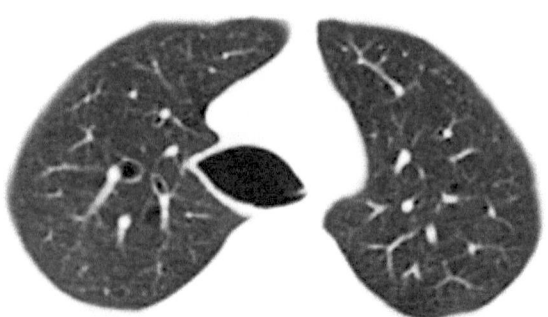

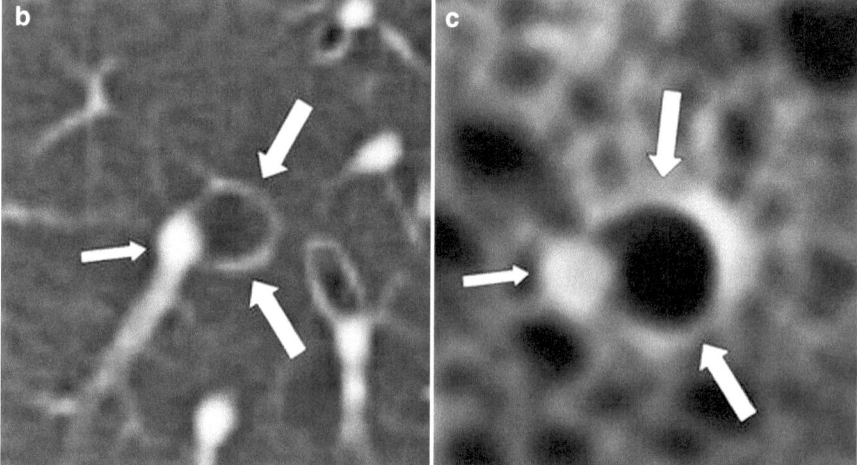

Fig. 4.76b, c Experimental model of enlarged bronchiole; the signet ring sign in the patient (**b**, *left image*) and the sponge (**c**, *right image*)

Potential differential diagnoses include the following:

- *Infectious* – viral, mycoplasmal, MAI, (Mycobacterium avium-intracellulare) fungal
- *Allergic* – hypersensitivity pneumonitis (HP): centrilobular nodules
- *Toxic* – especially: chlorine, phosgene, oxides of nitrogen
- *Post-transplant*
- *Idiopathic*

An overview of bronchiolar chest imaging patterns is available online at the Radiology Assistant website [10].

Case 4.21

Figure 4.77 is that of a 34-year-old male with cough and dyspnea and no history of occupational exposures.

Fig. 4.77a, b CXRs of
bronchiolar pattern
demonstrating a tracheogram
(an air-bronchogram of the
trachea) due to surrounding
airway opacities

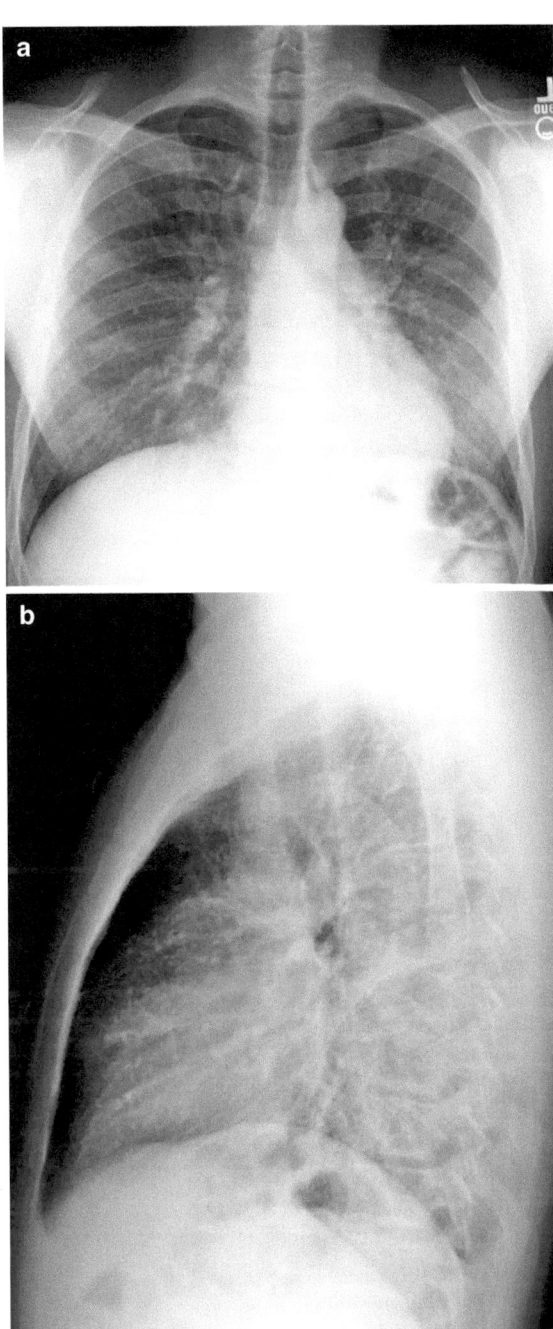

Fig. 4.77c, d HRCT of
above case showing diffuse
ground-glass and tree-in-bud
opacities with suggestion of
micronodules

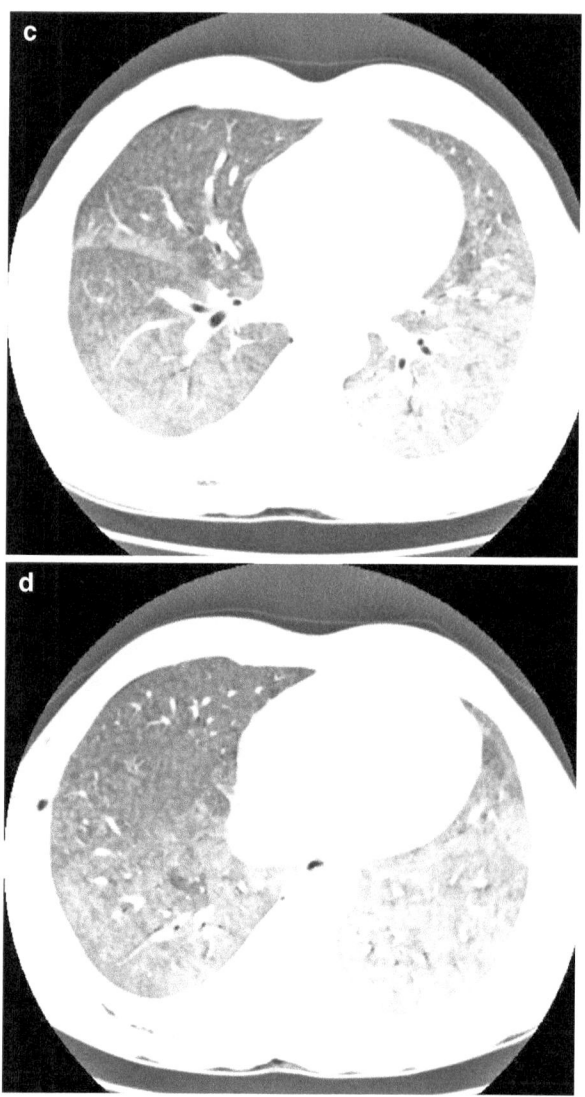

Findings: Bilateral, diffuse ground glass and scattered opacities causing a tracheogram (especially on left).

Pattern: Airway, specifically diffuse alveolar (centrilobular) nodular opacities. Other patterns considered: consolidative (alveolar opacities, however, can see vessels) and interstitial (nodular).

Differential
- Infectious – viral or atypical or idiopathic pneumonia
- Allergic – hypersensitivity pneumonitis
- Toxic
- Post-transplant

The following high resolution (HR) CT of the above case shows diffuse ground-glass and tree-in-bud opacities with a suggestion of micronodules.

Diagnosis: Extrinsic allergic alveolitis (Hypersensitivity pneumonitis)

One needs a high index of suspicion to narrow to this differential diagnosis. This emphasizes why a good occupational and/or hobby exposure history is necessary since this process often manifests subtle findings.

Etiology: Sensitization to repeated inhalational exposure of organic antigens. These organic antigens include a variety of sources (dairy, grain and wood products, animal dander or proteins, and water reservoir vaporizers). The most common

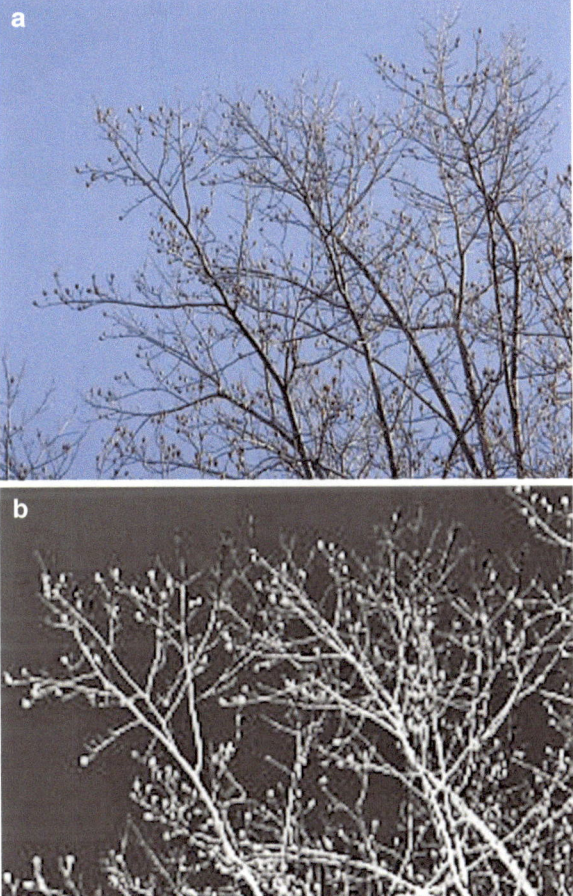

Fig. 4.78 (**a**, **b**) Demonstrates a color photograph of a tree-in-bud in the spring. This image was converted to black and white and inverted to help show CT findings (photo and processing by Dr. Folio). (**c**) This is a immunocompromised child with severe bronchiectasis and infectious bronchiolitis manifesting as centrilobular tree-in-bud opacities. (**d**) is a collage with the photo of an actual tree-in-bud, superimposed over the right lower lobe (*outlined in black rectangle*) to demonstrate similarity of the tree-in-bud finding and the origin of the term. Note how the blurry tree-in-bud in the patient (*dotted circle*) is similar in appearance to the imported photo

Fig. 4.78 (continued)

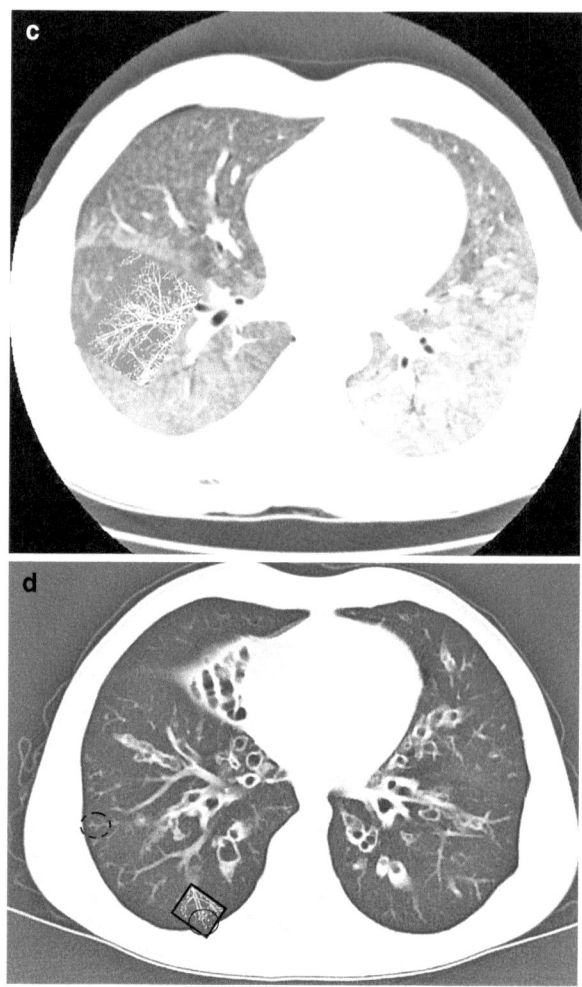

antigens are thermophilic actinomycetes and avian proteins. The most common diseases are farmer's lung and bird fancier's lung. Combination of clinical, radiographic, and pulmonary function tests. Bronchioalveolar lavage can suggest diagnosis. Biopsy may be needed in some cases. A great reference for HRCT findings is the University of California San Francisco Chest Primer [11].

The following should help the beginning radiology student to understand the tree-in-bud finding.

References

1. Feigin DS. A revised system for analysis of abnormal pulmonary images. Chest. 1993;103(2):594–600.
2. MacMahon H, Austin JHM, Gamsu G, Herold CJ, Jett JR, Naidich DP, et al. Guidelines for management of small pulmonary nodules detected on CT scans: a statement from the Fleischner Society. Radiology. 2005;237:395–400.
3. Yamamoto M, et. al. Quantitative Evaluation Method for Lung Tumor with Fractal Analysis of X-ray CT Images. For images of malignant and benign masses, go to. http://www.nirs.go.jp/report/nene/H10/1/003.html. Accessed 20 Oct 2011.
4. Shaffer K. Role of radiology for imaging and biopsy of solitary pulmonary nodules. Chest. 1999;116:519–22.
5. Slotto J, Folio L. Cystic fibrosis chest x-ray findings: a teaching analog. Mil Med Int J AMSUS. 2008;173(7):xii, xiii.
6. Dubois D. Miliary nodular INTERSTITIAL pattern (lung). http://rad.usuhs.edu/medpix/parent.php3?mode=display_factoid&recnum=841 Medpix. 2000. Accessed 20 Oct 2011.
7. Case study and photographs are used by permission, Shogan P, Muncy T, McCarthy K, Folio L. *Pneumocystis jiroveci* pneumonia. Mil Med Int J AMSUS. 2008;173(10):vii, viii.
8. National Heart Lung and Blood Institute. What is pulmonary arterial hypertension? http://www.nhlbi.nih.gov/health/health-topics/topics/pah
9. Broussard E. Pulmonary artery hypertension – shunt vascularity. In: MedPix. 2003. http://rad.usuhs.edu/medpix/radpix.html?mode=single&recnum=4854&table=&srchstr=&search#pic Accessed 20 Oct 2011.
10. Smithuis R, van Delden O, Schaefer-Prokop c. Radiology assistant. http://www.radiologyassistant.nl/en/42d94cd0c326b. Accessed 24 May 2011.
11. Webb R. The University of California San Francisco Chest Primer. http://pathhsw5m54.ucsf.edu/ctpath/ctpathcontents.html. Accessed 24 May 2011.
12. Folio LR. "Occupational Medicine Board Essentials." 2004.

Chapter 5
Abnormalities Involving the Pleura

Abnormalities involving the pleura include pathologic processes (masses, calcifications, infections, thickening) of the pleura, in addition to fluid and air collections within the pleural space. This chapter will start off with more common conditions such as pleural effusions and pneumothorax, followed by less common/ more complex processes.

Pleural Effusion

Definition: fluid in the potential space between the parietal and visceral pleura. This usually results in obliteration part or all of the hemidiaphragms (silhouette sign), blunting of the costophrenic angles both peripherally on the frontal projection and posteriorly on the lateral.

Case 5.1

Figure 5.1 demonstrates a left pleural effusion on interdepartmental PA and lateral, a portable projection on same patient next day, then on CT.

Technique and Positioning Revisited

In the Chap. 2 of this book, we reviewed how technical factors such as rotation, X-ray energy, and markers are important. The preceding and following examples of the appearance of effusion also demonstrate how technique, especially portable positioning, is important in evaluating effusions, and differentiating them from other conditions such as consolidations.

L.R. Folio, *Chest Imaging*, DOI 10.1007/978-1-4614-1317-2_5,

Fig. 5.1a,b PA (**a**) and lateral (**b**) erect projections of the chest demonstrate blunting of left costophrenic angle with a meniscus peripherally on the PA and posteriorly on the lateral (*arrows*). Also note the left PICC line with tip in SVC

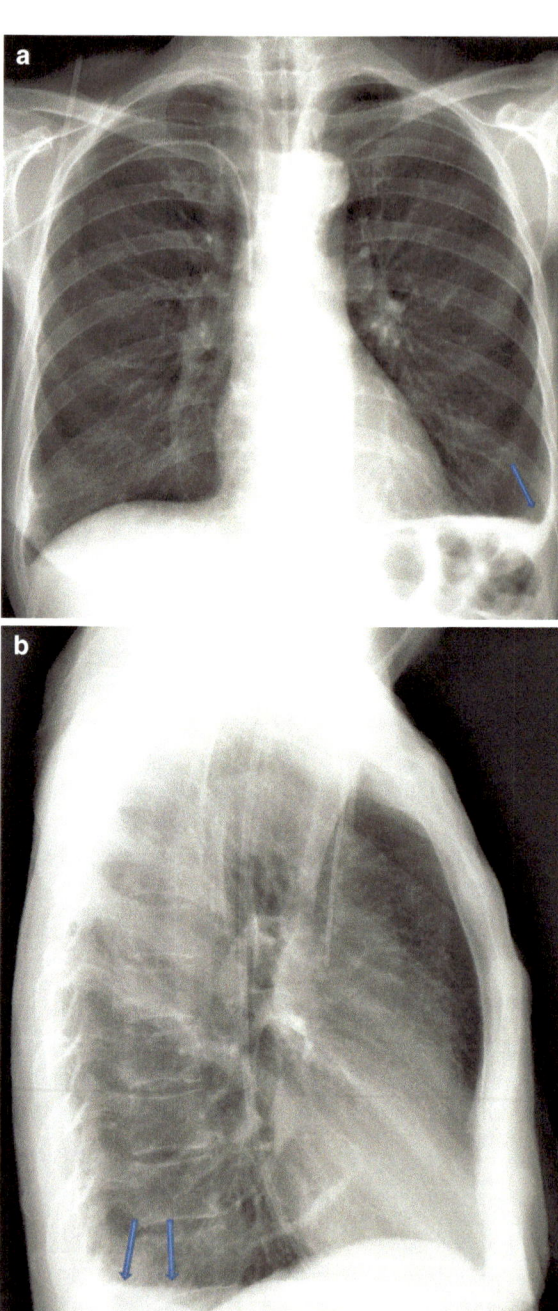

Fig. 5.1c Portable semi-erect AP projection (**c**) demonstrates a slightly larger left effusion on the same patient, next day. Note that the left hemidiaphragm is now totally obliterated, with a larger meniscus (*arrows*)

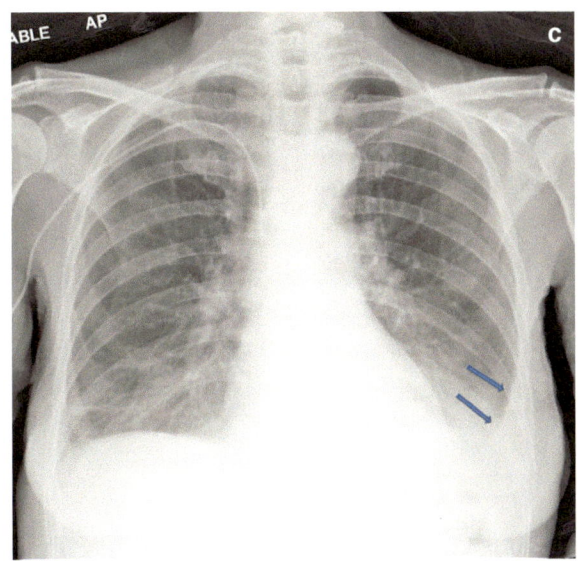

Fig. 5.1d Axial CT (**d**) of same patient showing left pleural effusion (*eff*), along with associated atelectasis (*atel*). The descending aorta is seen as "A"

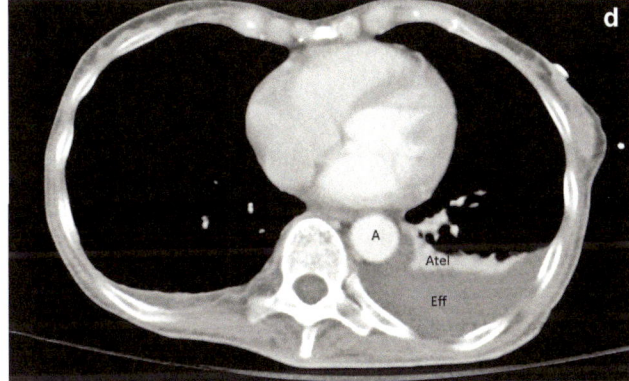

Case 5.2

See Fig. 5.2 for example of a positionally dependent effusion that is verified on the right side down (side down-side seen) decubitus projection (Fig. 5.2c).

Comparison of Effusions over Time

Optimally, portable images are obtained at similar angles each day, even if not erect, to allow accurate comparisons and assessment of change. To achieve this consistency, the technologist attempts the most upright projection, balanced with patient condition and ability to achieve this often impossible task. It is well documented that portable radiography of the chest is inconsistent and often inadequate [1, 2].

Fig. 5.2a PA projection
demonstrating blunting of
costophrenic angle with
associated opaque area (*dashed
circle*), with fluid tracking up
both minor fissure (*thin arrow*)
and major fissure (*wide arrow*)

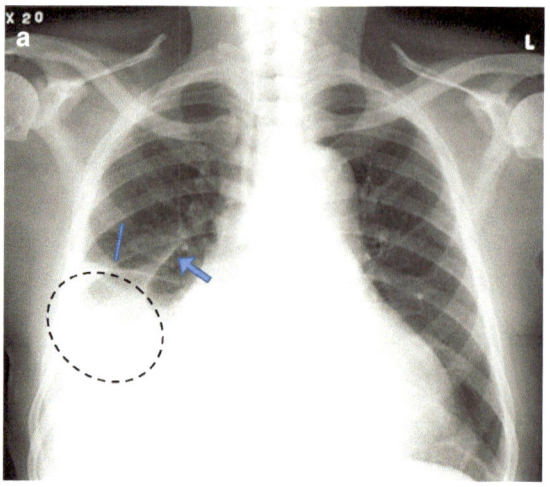

Fig. 5.2b Left side down
decubitus view fails to
demonstrate layering of effusion
in the left hemithorax. Any
layering of the right effusion is
not well demonstrated due to
overlying mediastinum

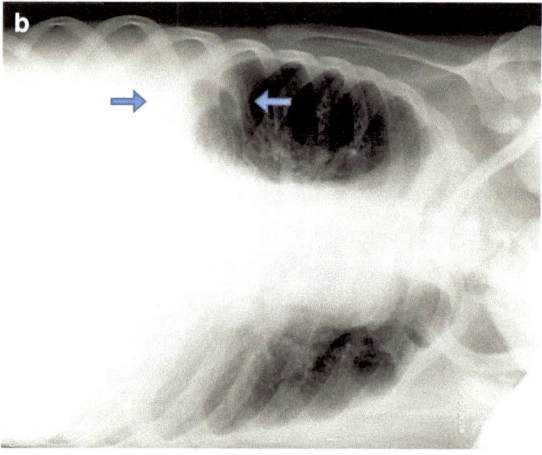

Fig. 5.2c This right side down
decubitus projection verifies that
the right effusion is positionally
dependent. This also helps to see
the extent of effusion since much
of the fluid seen on upright
projections is behind the
hemidiaphragm. One can
remember that with effusions and
what decubitus view to get: "side
down-side seen"

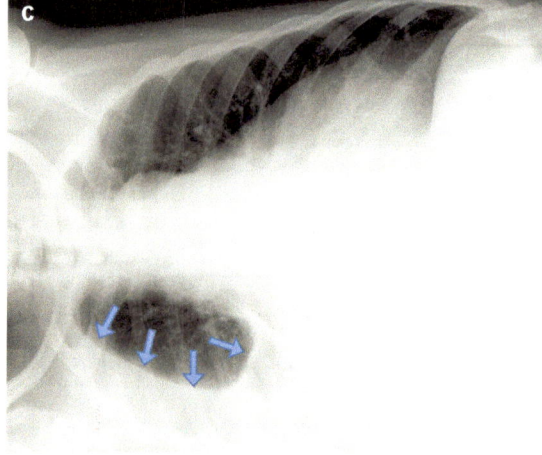

Evaluating the severity of effusions over time can be challenging, especially in the ICU, where exams on different days are at different inclinations (some supine, some nearly upright). The same effusion can look dramatically different in these two opposing positions.

Although devices have been used for years to attempt to demonstrate upright inclination, these only discern supine versus upright. A new device is being evaluated at NIH called the X-Clometer, that can quantify the degree of inclination (how upright is the projection?) to readily display the inclination [3].

See Fig. 5.3 for diagrams demonstrating how the simple X-Clometer works

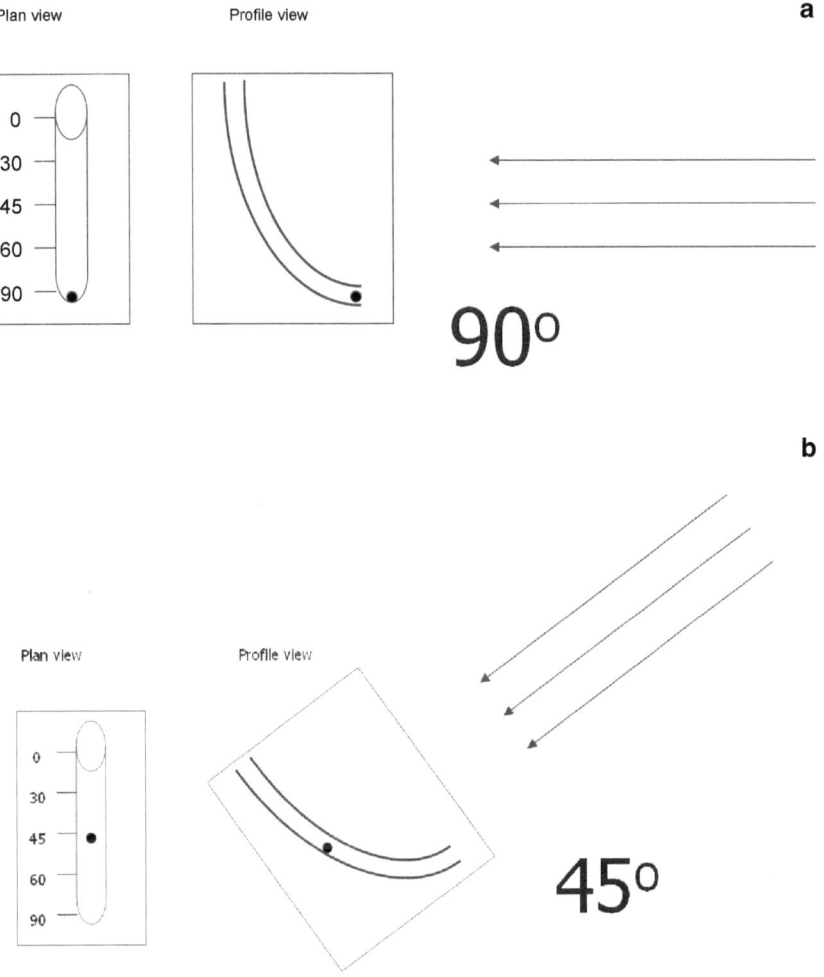

Fig. 5.3 This shows design and implementation of the X-Clometer with more accuracy than current markers. The *arrows* indicate the direction of the X-rays and the device is seen in profile (from the side of the cassette) and plan view (as seen on X-ray). These show the marker at 90° (*upright*, **a**), 45° (**b**), and 0° (*supine*, **c**)

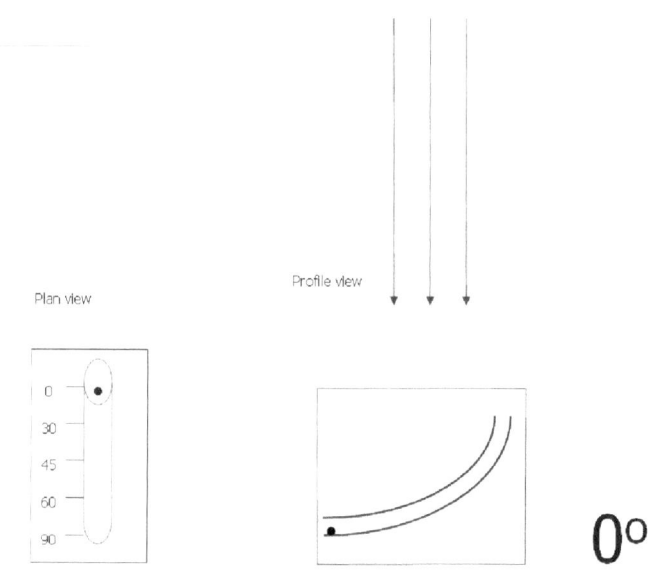

Plan view

Profile view

$0°$

Fig. 5.3 Continued

Loculated Fluid/Pseudotumor

Case 5.3

See Fig. 5.4 in a patient with both a peripheral loculated effusion and pseudotumor, or loculated fluid collection within a fissure.

Case 5.4

The following is a case where a young male was shot in the upper left chest by a sniper. More information can be obtained for a case report [4]. *Case and images reprinted with permission from Military Medicine: International Journal of AMSUS.*

Findings: Loss of left paratracheal stripe and pleural thickening consistent with pleural cap in upper lung field. In addition, left upper lung contusion and metallic fragmentation from bullet is noted.

Location: *Loculated pleural fluid*: blood from vascular injury.

Differential Diagnosis: Loculated blood in left upper pleural space.

Thickening

Pleural thickening can be a result of trauma, neoplasia, loculated fluid, inflammation, or chronic process such as connective tissue disease.

Fig. 5.4a Portable AP projection demonstrating right lower lung field opacity with meniscus and peripheral extension up to right lateral hemithorax (*Eff*) with rounded mass-like density in right mid lung field (*PsTum*) that is shown on CT (Fig. 5.4b) to represent a pseudotumor

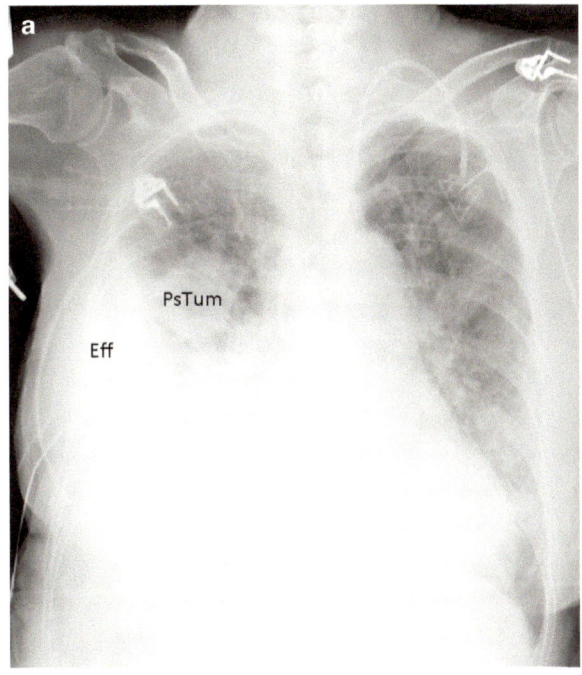

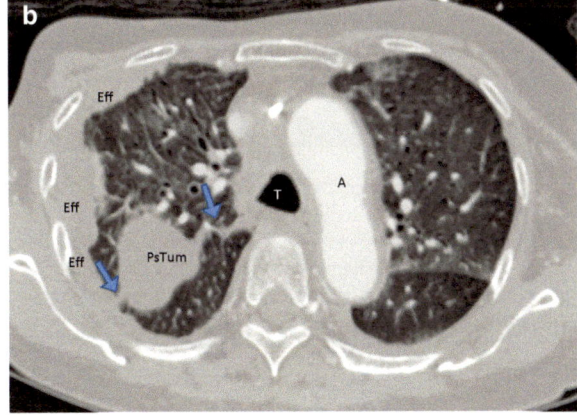

Fig. 5.4b Axial CT confirming partially loculated peripheral right pleural effusion (*eff*) and pseudotumor (*PsTum*) within the major fissure (*arrows*). Note also the trachea (*T*) and Aortic arch (*A*)

Fig. 5.4c Gunshot wound to the chest; note the "pleural cap" (fluid density capping the left apex) due to loculated hemothorax. This widens the left paratracheal stripe we learned about earlier. Also note linear consolidation of left upper lung field due to wound path

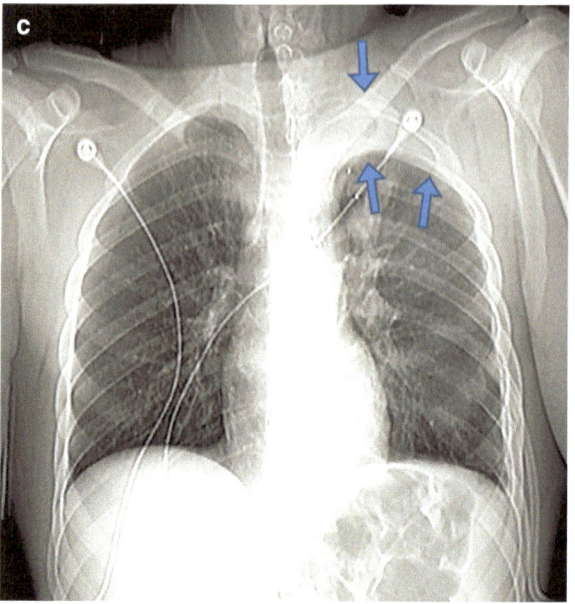

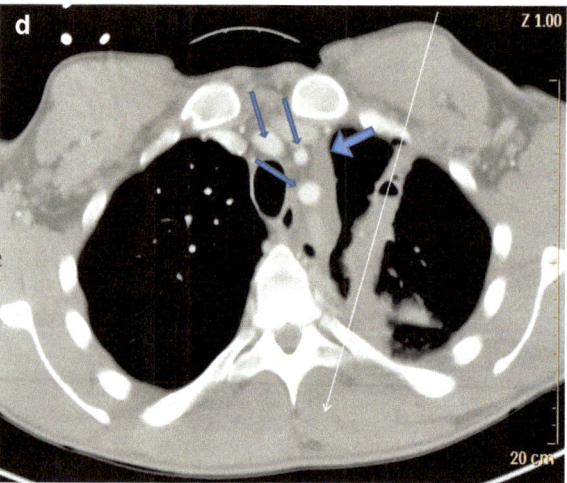

Fig. 5.4d Gunshot wound on CT confirming the wound path (permanent/temporary cavity filled with blood). The *white arrow* demonstrates the wound path; note the contused/lacerated lung along the path. This is a para-axial CT post IV contrast, confirming an angle compatable with a sniper shot. The *wide arrow* highlights the hemothorax (loculated effusion) that represents the pleural cap. The *small arrows* demonstrate the major arterial branches from the aorta on the left (right brachiocephalic, left subclavian, and common carotid arteries and left brachiocephalic vein)

Pneumothorax

The following example, which shows a pneumothorax, is the case of a patient who presented with chest pain. See Fig. 5.5a and b for what to look for in the search pattern presented earlier in this book. Also see the next section showing a model of pneumothorax using a wine glass with a balloon.

The following visual analogies depict pneumothorax, pleural effusion without pneumothorax, and hydropneumothorax. The photos are by Dr. Les Folio.

The side-by-side images in the following figures depict the air present when pneumothorax occurs. In the image on the left, the air between the glass and balloon is analogous to a pneumothorax.

Fluid and Air

Hydropneumothorax (or hemopneumothorax) is a combination of pleural fluid and pneumothorax. A straight air-fluid level, as seen in Fig. 5.6, differentiates this entity from pleural effusion without pneumothorax. Effusions without pneumothorax have a meniscus as we have seen.

The following case is of a blast injury to the chest resulting in a traumatic hemopneumothorax. More details about this case and the analogous models are available online [5].

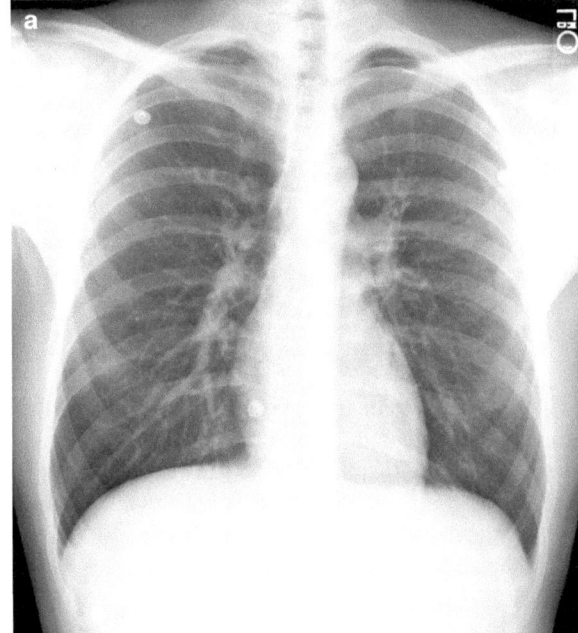

Fig. 5.5a CXR with subtle left apical pneumothorax

Fig. 5.5b Close-up of CXR in same patient with *arrows* pointing to a small pneumothorax in the left apex

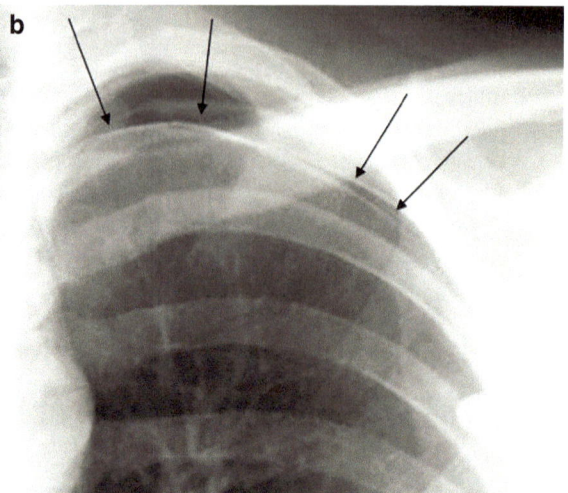

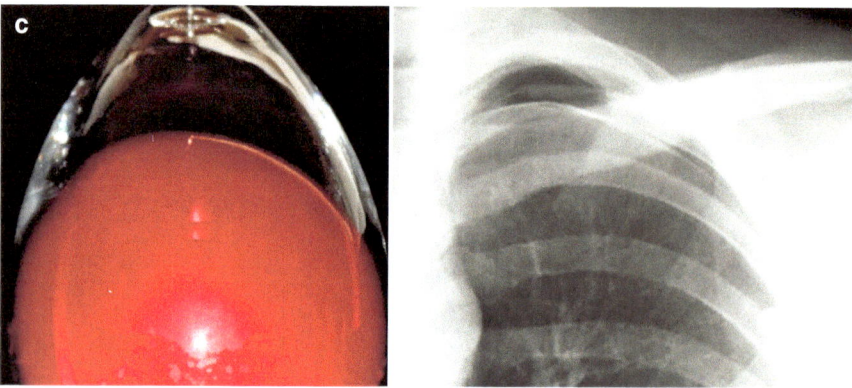

Fig. 5.5c Balloon (incompletely filling glass) in wine glass (*left*) analog to pneumothorax (*right*). The partially filled balloon is analogous to a partial deflated lung. The space between the balloon and the glass contains air, similar to the potential pleural space when occupied by air

Analogous Model

The side-by-side images (Fig. 5.6b, c) depict the balloon analog of hydropneumothorax [1]. In both images, the arrows point to the meniscus, which is typical on lateral pleural effusion. *Meniscus in wine glass (left) analog to meniscus in CXR.* The straight air-fluid level that is not possible when pneumothorax is not present. Also, note that the space between the chest wall (the glass) and the lung (the balloon) is occupied by both air and fluid.

Fig. 5.6a Blast exposed combat casualty showing fluid and air in this erect projection. (Case and images reprinted with permission from Military Medicine: International Journal of AMSUS)

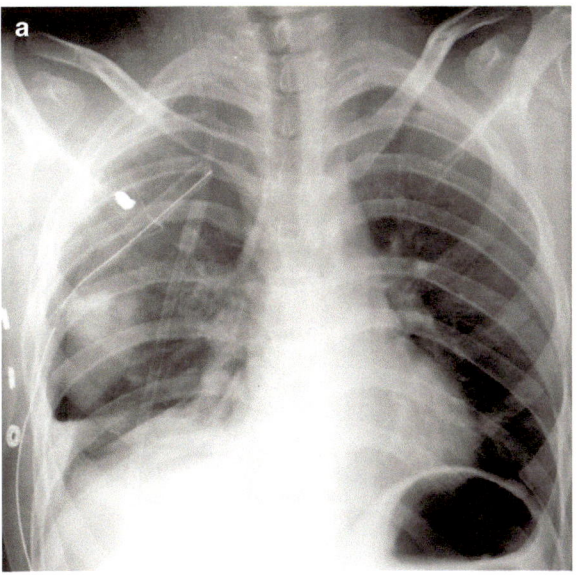

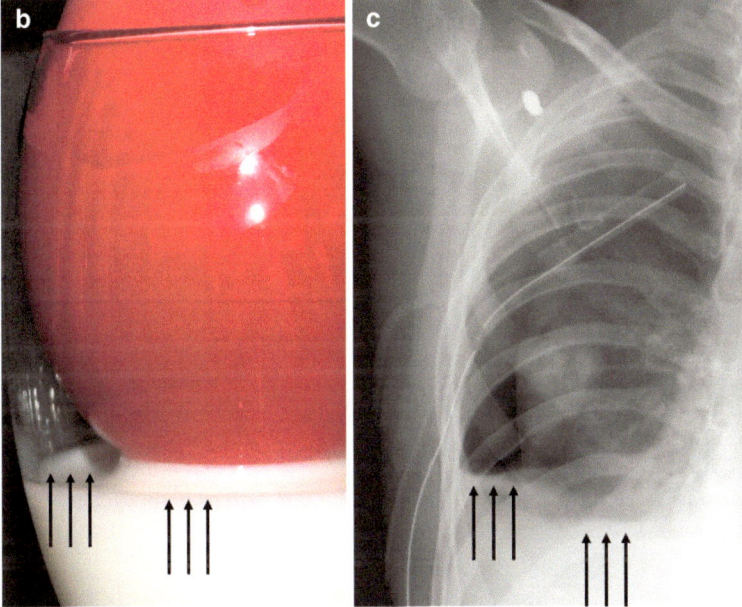

Fig. 5.6b,c Balloon analog (**b**) showing milk layer and partially filled balloon (lung). The photo was taken with camera alignment parallel to floor (perpendicular to gravity) representing an erect projection. Note similarity with actual hydropneumothorax (**c**). The *arrows* demonstrate how fluid level can be perceived in several layers

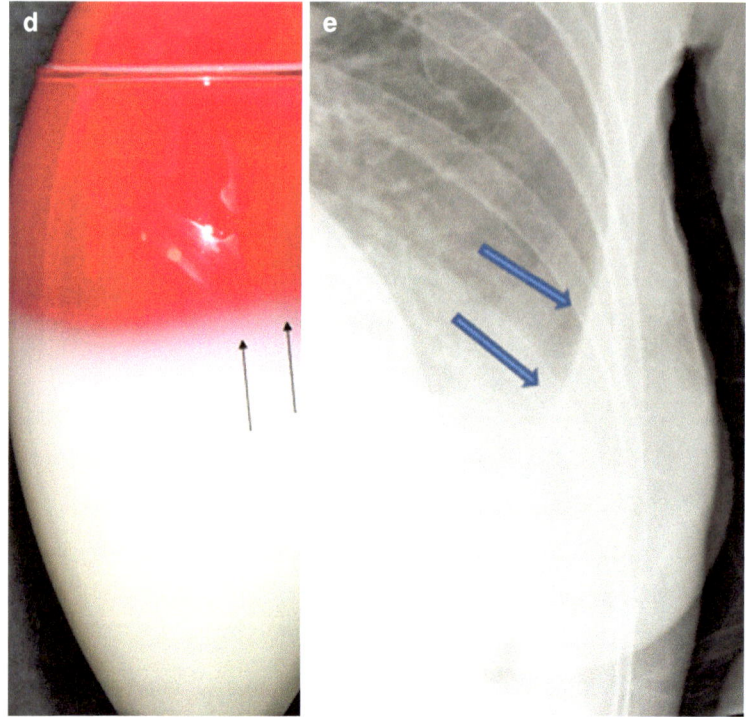

Fig. 5.6d,e Recall case 5.1 with the left pleural effusion and meniscus. This balloon/glass analogy with the balloon filling the glass demonstrates how the milk is compressed against the glass, making a meniscus-like configuration

Calcified Plaque

The following example is the case of a 77-year-old male retired factory worker seen for follow-up.

Findings: Partially well-marginated calcific opacity left upper lung field.

Location: Lateral confirms peripheral location such as pleura (calcified plaque).

Differential Diagnosis: Calcified pleural plaque of asbestos-related disease.

Figure 5.7c is the axial view on CT.

Fig. 5.7a Pleural calcified
plaque on PA (*dotted oval*)

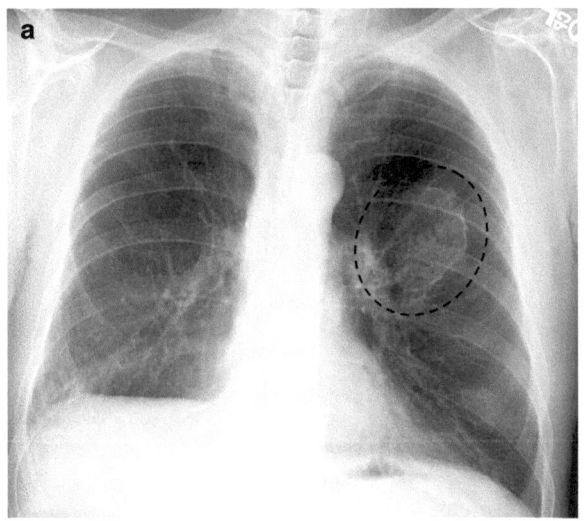

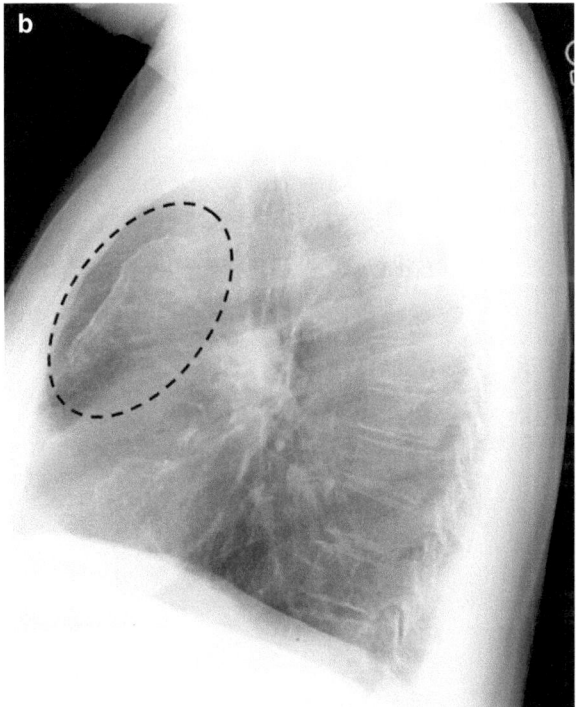

Fig. 5.7b Pleural calcified
plaque on lateral (*dotted oval*)

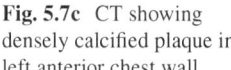

Fig. 5.7c CT showing densely calcified plaque in left anterior chest wall

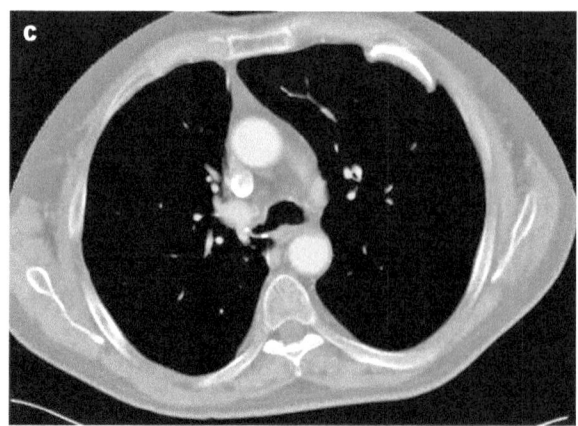

References

1. Wandtke JC. Bedside chest radiography. Radiology. 1994;190:1–10 [PMID: 8043058].
2. Bekemeyer WB et al. Efficacy of chest radiography in a respiratory intensive care unit. A prospective study. Chest. 1985;88(5):691–6 [PMID: 4053711].
3. Folio LR, Folio LS. X-Clometer: a device to measure inclination on portable radiographs. U.S. Provisional Application No. 61/452,364 filed March 14, 2011. HHS Reference No. E-036–2011/0.
4. Folio L, Robinson D. Apical hemothorax from Gunshot wound producing a Pleural Cap. Mil Med. 2009;174(12):xxiv–xxv.
5. Reed A, Dent M, Lewis S, Shogan P, Folio L. Hydropneumothorax. Mil Med. 2010;175(08): 625–6. http://rad.usuhs.edu/amsus.html. Accessed 24 May 2011.

Chapter 6
Abnormal Mediastinum

Abnormalities localized to the mediastinum include mass, enlargement, fluid, or air. For a brief description and graphic of the normal mediastinum CXR, see the mediastinal anatomy in chapter 3.

Mediastinal masses and other abnormalities occur in areas defined by anterior, middle, or posterior [1].

Each region has its own unique differential diagnosis, with some overlap such as vascular abnormalities. The other pages in the "Mediastinum" section of this book describe a method of systematically identifying abnormalities of the mediastinum, localizing more specifically, and provide simple mnemonics for recalling differentials in each region.

Radiological signs: Any disturbance of previously described mediastinal lines or edges could indicate an abnormality of the mediastinum.

Mechanism: Mass or other process can occur from many processes, depending on the anatomy in each area. Since vessels are in all three anatomic locations, tortuous or anomalous vessels can be included in each differential presented. Like with lung patterns, keep in mind that "mass" is a radiological finding and not synonymous with tumor. For example, a mass-like finding could be an aortic aneurism or enlarged pulmonary artery.

Anterior Mediastinal Mass

The anterior mediastinal region includes the following:

- Anterior to trachea, aorta, and arch vessels; superior to the pericardium; and is posterior to sternum. It contains fat, thymic remnants, internal mammary vessels, and lymph nodes.

L.R. Folio, *Chest Imaging*, DOI 10.1007/978-1-4614-1317-2_6,

You can use the six "T"s to help you remember the causes of anterior mediastinal masses.

- Thyroid lesions
- Thymic lesions (and parathyroid masses)
- Teratomas (and other germ cell tumors, see below mnemonic)
- "Terrible" lymphoma (Lymphadenopathy)
- Tortuous vessels (dissecting aorta, right arch)
- Trauma

To take this a step further, you can use the mnemonic YES CT to help you remember the types of germ cell tumors (under Teratoma, above). Some use ChESTY instead of YES CT.

Y – Yolk Sac
E – Endodermal Sinus Tumor (Yolk Sac)
S – Seminoma
C – Choriocarcinoma
T – Teratoma (most common in chest)

Case 6.1

Figure 6.1 is that of a 22-year-old active duty Marine Corps female smoker with chronic persistent cough and scattered wheezes. There was no significant medical or family history.

Findings: Well-rounded opacity overlying lateral left margin of the aorta and pulmonary artery. On lateral there is filling-in of the usually dark area behind the sternum (sometimes called RSCS or the RetroSternal Clear Space). Note that there are also calcifications in the mass.

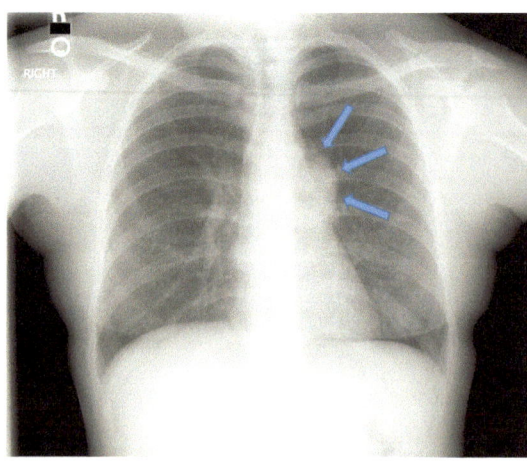

Fig. 6.1a Left hilar mass on PA (*arrows*). Note the hilar overlay sign (non-obliteration of aorta or main pulmonary artery)

Fig. 6.1b Mass on lateral anteriorly located
(*large arrows*), note absence of RSCS and calcifications
(*small arrows*)

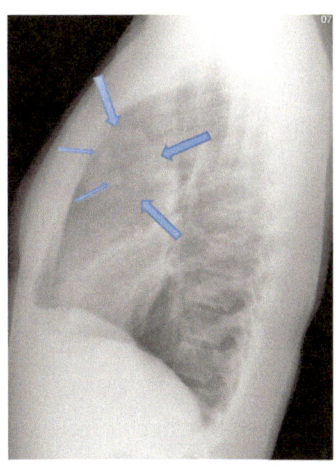

Fig. 6.1c CT of the same patient,
which reveals a mass (*arrows*) in
the anterior mediastinum. In the
soft tissue window on the right,
note the fat density as well as
calcification representing a tooth

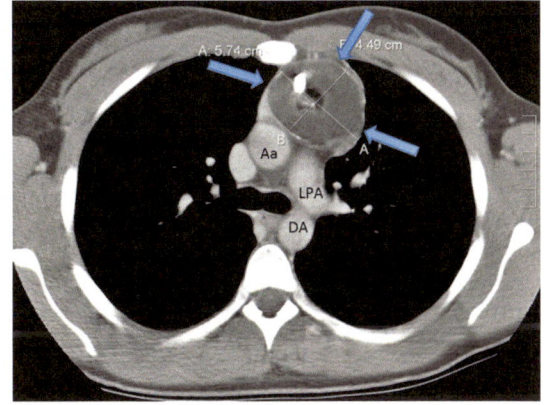

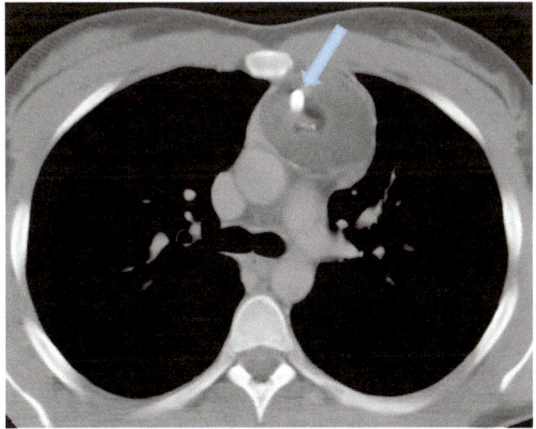

Fig. 6.1d Axial CT bone
algorithm highlighting tooth
morphology (*arrow*)

Location: Anterior mediastinum.

Differential Diagnosis: Because of the calcifications and well-roundedness, the differential was narrowed down to teratoma (to include germ cell tumors) and was surgically confirmed.

Teratoma is the most common anterior mediastinal germ cell tumor. The incidence in males is equal to the incidence in females, and there is a bimodal age distribution (infancy and 20–40 year olds). The majority of patients are asymptomatic at the time of diagnosis.

- Teratoma Pathology
- Teratomas contain tissue from at least two primitive germ layers (endoderm, mesoderm, ectoderm).
- Approximately 50–75% have little to no malignant potential.
- Types of teratoma include mature, immature, and malignant.
- The treatment is typically surgical excision.

Middle Mediastinal Mass

The middle mediastinal region includes the following:

- Contains the pericardium and its contents, brachiocephalic vessels, ascending and transverse aorta, SVC and IVC, phrenic nerves, upper portion of vagus nerve, pulmonary arteries and veins, trachea and main bronchi, and their contiguous lymph nodes.

You can use the mnemonic LATTE to remember the following masses/conditions of the middle mediastinum. Although the esophagus is not in the middle mediastinum by definition, it is included for two reasons: esophageal tumors can extend into the middle mediastinum, and most importantly, it makes the mnemonic work!

L – Lymph nodes, metastasis
A – Aorta (and other vascular lesions)
T – Trachea, bronchi, bronchogenic cyst, inlet lesions
T – Tumor
E – Esophagus: carcinoma, hiatal hernia, duplication Cysts

The more specific differential of these anatomic regions includes the following:

- Lymph nodes
- Lymph node enlargement (most are malignant)
  - Adenopathy
    - Neoplastic adenopathy
    - Inflammatory adenopathy
    - Sarcoid; Castleman's disease
    - Inhalational Disease adenopathy

Posterior Mediastinal Mass

The middle mediastinal region includes the following:
*   Bounded anteriorly by the pericardium and vertical portion of diaphragm, later-ally by the mediastinal pleura, and posteriorly by the thoracic vertebrae. It con-tains the esophagus, descending aorta, azygous and hemiazygous veins, thoracic duct, autonomic nerves, fat, and lymph nodes.

There are a number of causes of posterior mediastinal masses. You can use the mnemonic NECO to help you remember the overall differential.

N – Neurogenic
*   Nerve root tumors
*   Ganglion tumors
*   Paragangliomas
*   Lateral meningocele

E – Esophageal
*   Esophageal carcinoma
*   Benign esophageal neoplasm
*   Hiatal hernia
*   Pulsion diverticuli
*   Achalasia
*   Esophageal varices

C – Cysts
*   Duplication cysts
*   Enteric cysts
*   Neurenteric cysts
*   Bronchogenic cysts

O – Others
*   Extralobar sequestration – 2/3 in lower lobes
*   Inflammation
*   Vascular lesions
*   Trauma
*   Abdominal origin posterior masses, e.g., Bochdalek hernia

---

Case 6.2

Figure 6.2 show CXRs demonstrating a partially circumscribed mass

The Fig. 6.2c is a CT of the same patient showing an irregular mass emanating from the esophagus, consistent with an esophageal stromal tumor (confirmed by surgery).

Fig. 6.2a Subtle mediastinal mass in the left medial chest, adjacent to the descending aortic edge

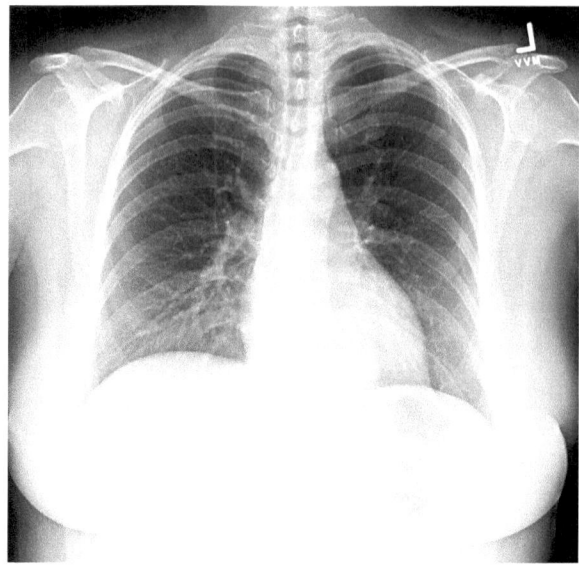

Fig. 6.2b Posterior mediastinal mass circled

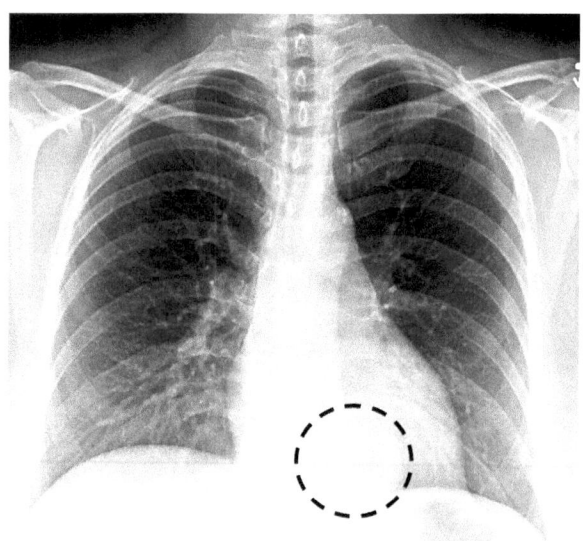

Mediastinal Enlargement

The mediastinum can be enlarged from mass; however, one should also consider vessels, blood, or fluid. See Fig. 6.3 for CXR and CT of enlarged irregular mediastinum compatible with a ruptured aortic aneurism.

Fig. 6.2c Mediastinal mass
confirmed posterior and
esophageal on CT. The low
density mass is between the
descending aorta and the
heart

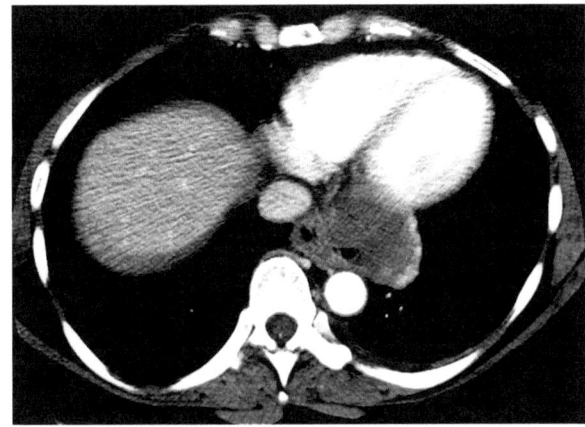

Fig. 6.3a This portable CXR
demonstrated a widened
mediastinum

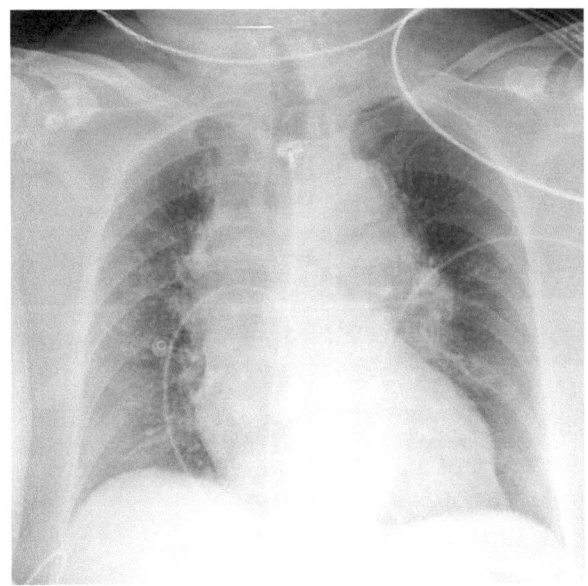

Case 6.3

The CXR in Fig. 6.3 is a case of a 50-year-old presenting with acute chest pain.

Findings: AP chest demonstrates grossly widened and ill-defined mediastinum.
Of note, the aortic calcification is not seen in the periphery of the aortic knob, indicating bleeding outside the aorta.

Location: Anterior middle and posterior mediastinum.

Fig. 6.3b Same image, now with *arrows* (*large*) highlighting the widened mediastinum. Note the aortic calcifications (*small arrows*) that are usually on the periphery of the aortic knob on the CXR

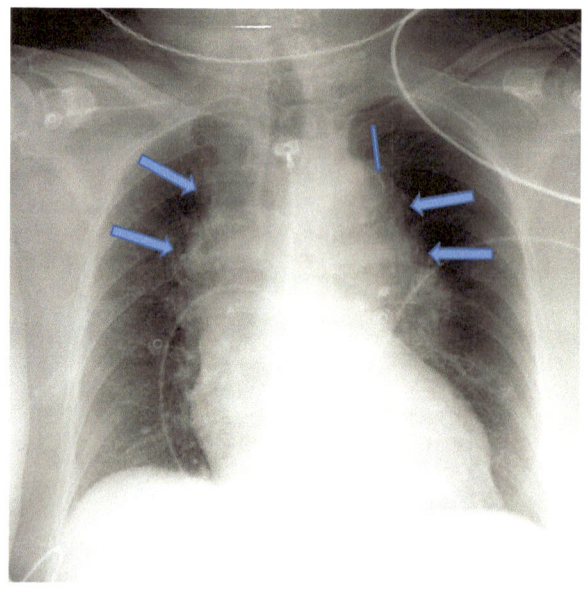

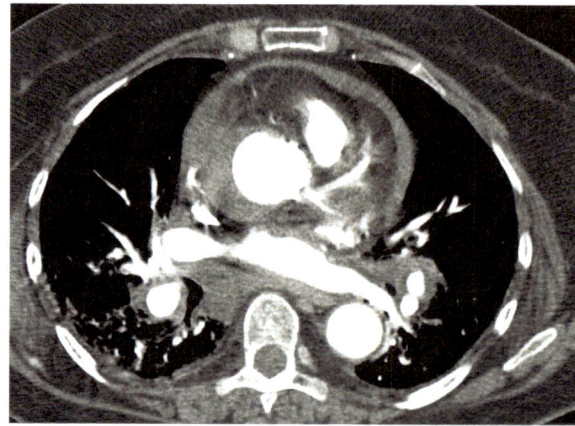

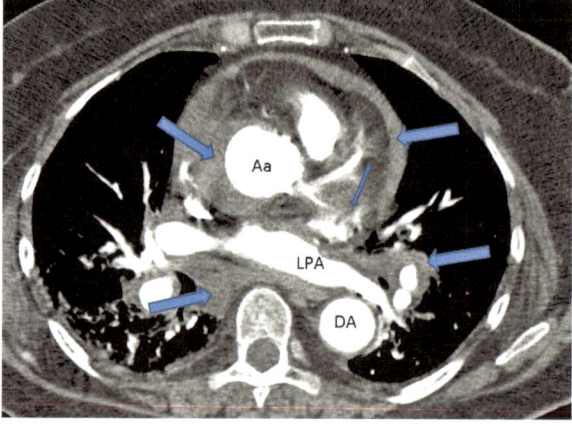

Fig. 6.3c An emergently ordered axial CT of the same patient and shows the active bleeding (*small arrows* on **d**) and less acute blood (*large arrows*) causing the widening seen on the CXR

Differential Diagnosis: Since this does not appear like mass and is lobulated and widely distributed, bleeding is first on the differential.
Diagnosis: Aortic rupture.

Reference

1. Zylak CM, Standen JR, Barnes GR, Zylak CJ. Pneumomediastinum revisited. Radiographics. 2000;20(4):1043–57.

Chapter 7
Abnormal Bones, Soft Tissue, and Other Findings

There are times when pathological processes occur outside the lungs and mediastinum, i.e., in the chest wall, to include bones and soft tissues. This is why we include these structures on the search pattern, in that one must think about those structures separately to deduce their potential involvement. I will also include a short synopsis of lines and tubes often seen in the ICU; they are easier to navigate than most think.

Mechanism: An abnormal process of the bones or soft tissues seen on the CXR, excluding lungs, mediastinum, and vascular structures already presented.

Case 7.1

The example case Fig. 7.1a-f highlights the thought process to include those processes that occur outside the lungs. This is the case of a 24-year-old male US Marine with posterior chest wall/rib pain for 4–6 months, increased with deep inspiration. This case will also point out a few signs and fundamentals presented earlier in the book. This case is reprinted with permission from: Warnock et al. (2008) [1].

Findings: Poorly marginated opacity overlying right hila. On the lateral CXR, a partially marginated opacity is noted posteriorly.

Location/Pattern: The posterior location raises possibilities such as pleural based (since the obtuse angles posteriorly) or bone origin.

Differential Diagnosis: Because of the location and characteristics, it is best to approach this CXR by analyzing it based on broad possibilities: posterior lung mass (or focal consolidation), pleural-based mass or process, or bone process.

Posterior lung mass would include the lung mass pattern and posterior mediastinal differential.

L.R. Folio, *Chest Imaging*, DOI 10.1007/978-1-4614-1317-2_7,   131
© Henry M. Jackson Foundation for the Advancement of Military Medicine, Inc. 2012

Fig. 7.1a PA CXR
demonstrating an ill-defined right
hilar mass. Note the hilar overlay
sign and boney destruction (see
also Fig. 7.1c)

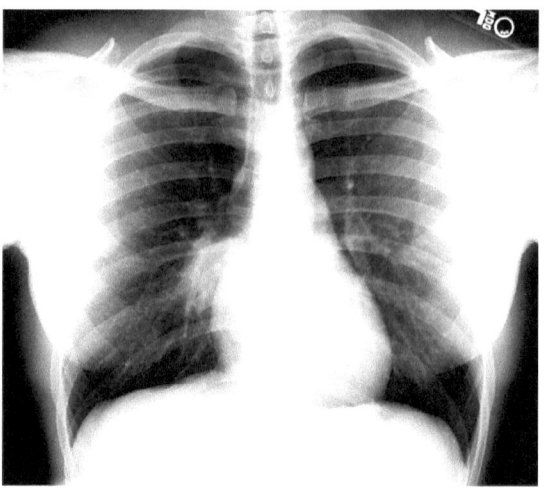

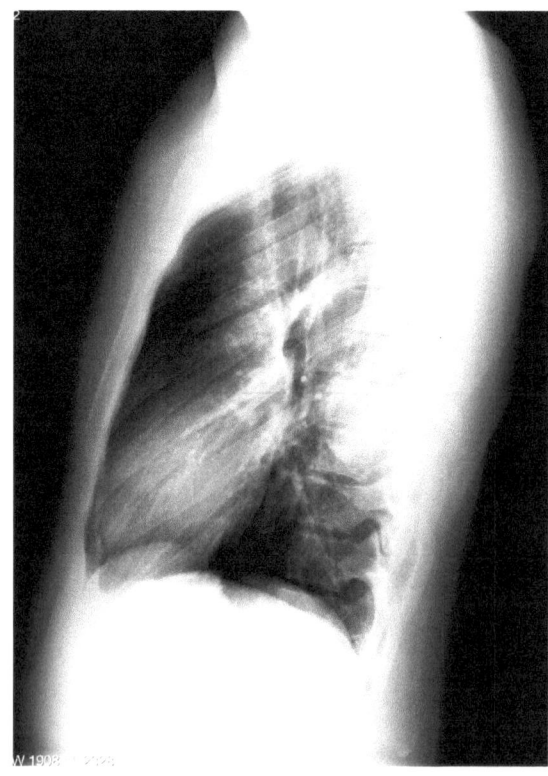

Fig. 7.1b Lateral CXR showing
a positive spine sign/opacity
posteriorly with obtuse angled
margins superiorly and inferiorly

Fig. 7.1c Thoracic spine plain radiograph better demonstrating bone destruction. Note the absence of medial right 9th rib (*wide arrow*) and moth-eaten T9 vertebral body on right (*thin arrow*)

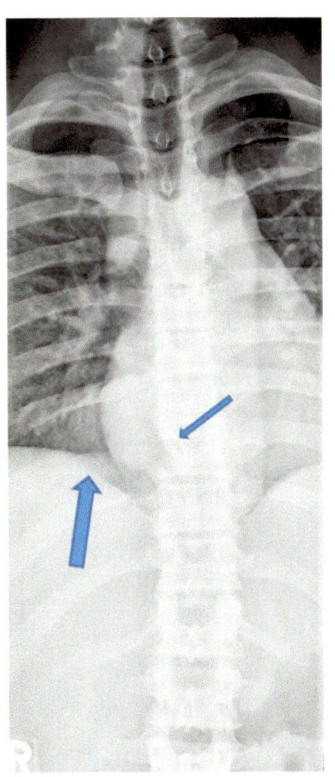

Pleural based masses
- Solitary pleural density
- Loculated pleural effusion
- Mesothelioma
- Metastases
- Splenosis

Bone process
- Benign primary bone tumors include the following:
  - Chondroblastoma
  - Chondromyxoid fibroma
  - Osteochondroma
  - Giant cell
  - Enchondroma
  - Fibrodysplasia

- Malignant primary bone tumors include the following:
  - Chondrosarcoma
  - Osteoblastoma, aggressive variant
  - Osteosarcoma

Fig. 7.1d PA CXR with
arrows pointing to the mass

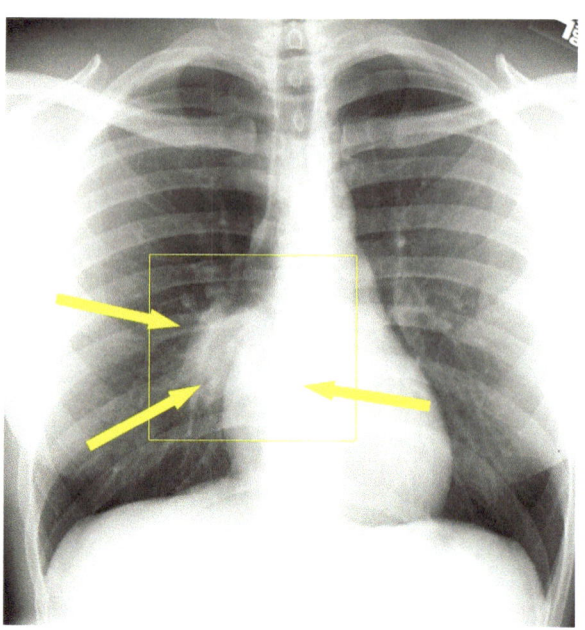

Fig. 7.1e Lateral CXR with *arrows* pointing to the
mass

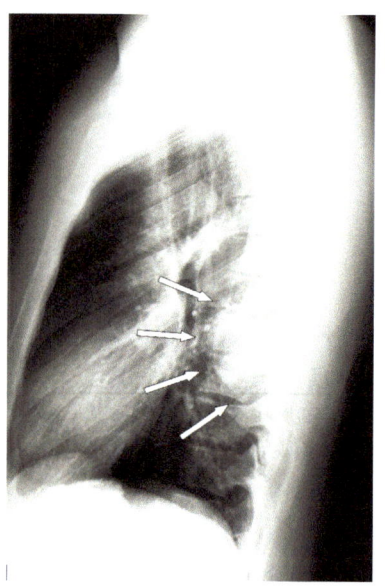

Diagnosis: This turned out to be a chondroblastoma with secondary aneurysmal
bone cyst. Although this differential diagnosis is unusual, the point here is to use search
pattern considerations of structures and regions other than lung and mediastinum.

Figure 7.1d–f show a large, ill-defined, lobulated mass located in the right
paraspinal region in this patient.

Fig. 7.1f Chondroblastoma on CT. Note the rib and spinal element destruction. Inclusion of two adjacent bones enters the infection differential

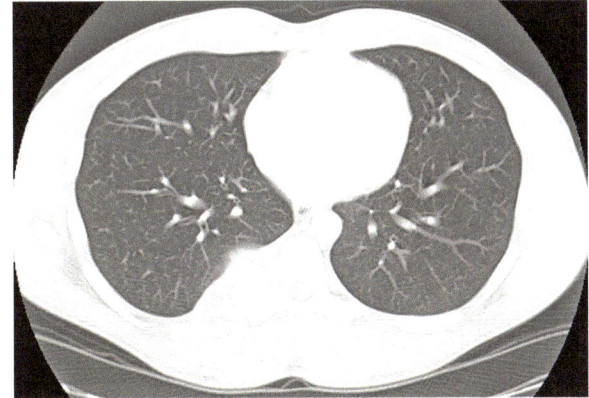

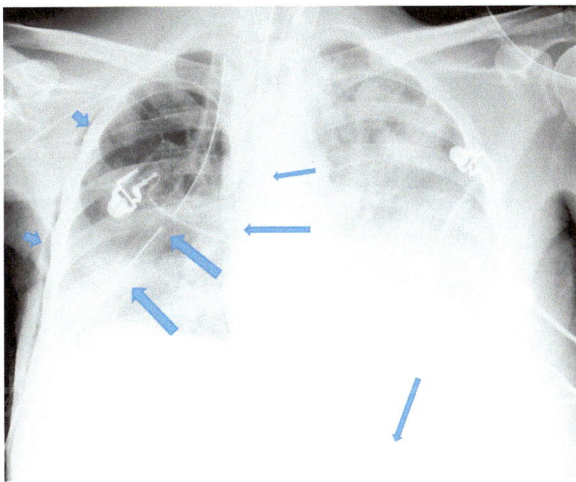

Fig. 7.2a This ICU patient has the ET tube a bit close to carina for my liking (within one cm; *thinnest arrow* near carina). The PICC line is seen entering from the right arm and entering the right brachycephalic, terminating (the tip) in the SVC (*long arrow* overlying mediastinum). A right chest tube is noted (*widest arrows*) with sideport (most *superior arrow*) and with tip in right apex. Subcutaneous emphysema is noted lateral to the ribs in the chest wall soft tissues (*shortest arrows*). NG tube is seen in stomach (*long arrow* over stomach)

Lines and Tubes

Several figures have included lines and tubes throughout this book. Please refer back to the abnormal parenchyma chapter, for example, placements of chest and ET (EndoTracheal Tubes), PICC, Port-a-Cath, IJ, and other central lines.

See Fig. 7.2a for many of the common lines found in typical ICUs.

See Fig. 7.2b for a more worrisome picture of a failed right jugular line placement with a bleed into the right hemithorax. Also the ET tube was to distal, in the Right Mainstem Bronchus.

Fig. 7.2b Example of a failed right jugular line placement with a bleed into the right hemithorax (*wide short arrows*). The ET tube was to the distal, in the right mainstem bronchus (*long arrow*). This causes further decreased aeration to the right lung (shut off from bypassing only aerating left lung). PICC line coming from right arm is okay in SVC (*wide arrow*). Also NG tube is okay coiled in stomach. Remainder of lines are ECG lines on patient

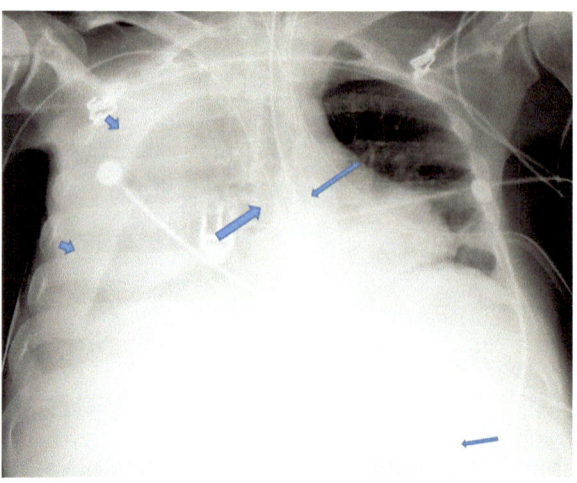

Fig. 7.2c Note the left IJ line (*long arrow*) enters brachiocephalic, then takes a turn to the left jugular (*short arrow* in left neck). The ET is a few centimeters above the carina (*long wide arrow*) and the NG tube is within the stomach (*short arrow* overlying stomach)

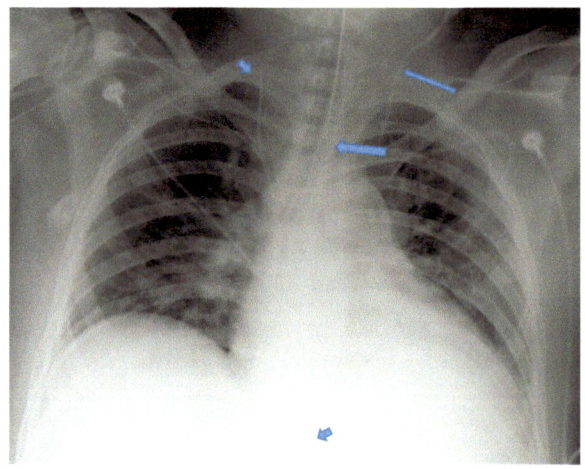

Figure 7.2c demonstrates how lines can go in many directions; to no fault of the faculty, staff, interns, residents, and fellows that place them. Malplacement is exactly why routine chest images are obtained.

One helpful tool I have used to help locate lines is by reversing the grayscale. A better recently development is called Tube and Line Visualization Software by Carestream Health (Rochester, NY). [2] that increases conspicuity of radiopaque devices (see Fig. 7.2d, e).

With portable DR (Direct Radiography) and instant viewing, ICU and other providers can instantly see their tube placements, now digitally enhanced to save trips to the PACS and/or radiology department. Also avoids waiting for a report or a call for a misplaced line or tube. Nonradiologists seem to favor the digitally enhanced

Fig. 7.2d,e This patient has a left-sided Swan catheter (too far lateral, should be a few centimeters from midline) in the right pulmonary artery, in addition to a right PICC line and ET tube (*arrows*). Note the lower image demonstrating increased conspicuity of the lines and tubes (special line and tube enhancement sofware). Also note the diffuse patchy airspace opacities that represented edema in this patient. The left hemidiaphragm is not well visualized, indicating effusion in this case

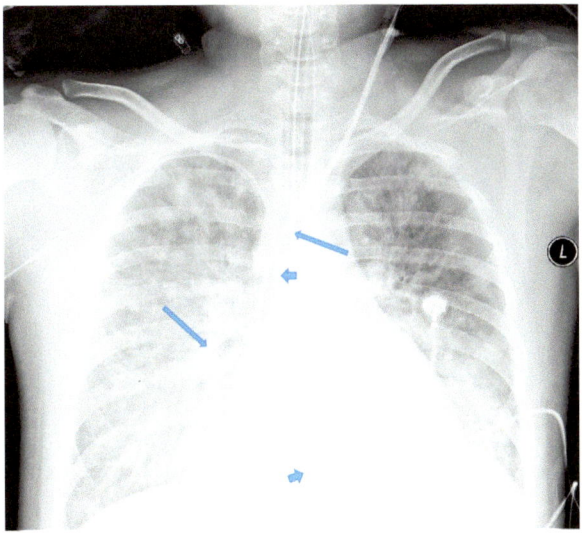

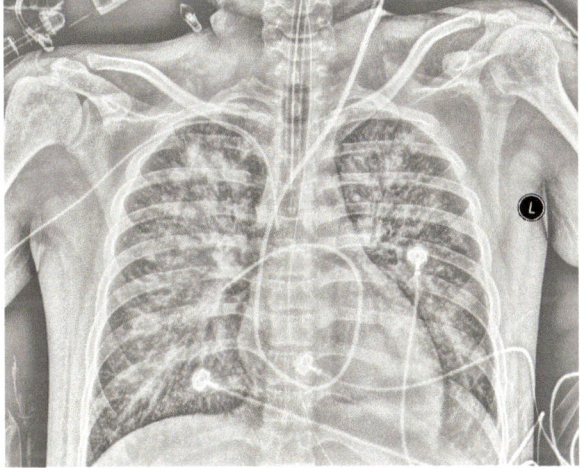

images. I call this process "digital solarization" as it is similar to what we used to do in the darkroom by turning the lights on halfway through development.

Another trick for quickly assessing for rib fractures is to invert the CXR; they stand out because our usual eye scanning is thrown off.

Lastly, do not forget to look at the abdomen as it is partially included in every CXR. See this last case where the patient also had a SBO (Small Bowel Obstruction).

Figure 7.3a and b highlights a few basic points. Look everywhere (the search pattern); think about everything (within reason, but region and pattern approach). This last case is a surgical emergency and must be recognized. When in doubt, get additional films and call someone more experienced than you.

Fig. 7.3a Note the distended small bowel loops in the upper abdomen. This turned out to be an SBO (see Fig. 7.3b)

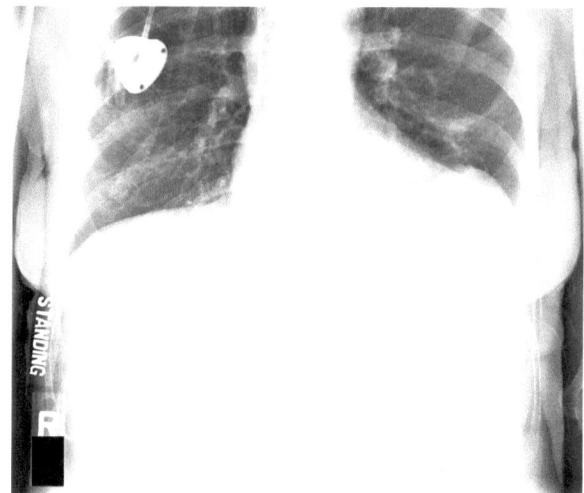

Fig. 7.3b Note diffusely dilated small bowel loops. No large bowel loops are seen

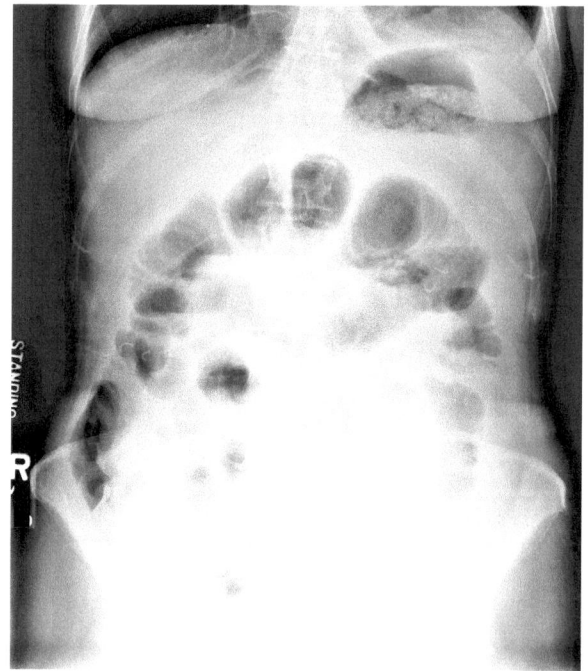

References

1. Warnock A, Gibson M, Folio L. Chondroblastoma with secondary aneurysmal bone cyst. Mil Med Int J AMSUS. 2008;173(2):xiii–xiv.
2. Foos DH, Yankelevitz DF, Wang X, Berlin D, Zappetti D, Cham M, Sanders A, Parker KN, Henschke CI. Improved visualization of tubes and lines in portable intensive care unit radiographs: a study comparing a new approach to the standard approach. Clinical Imaging. 2011;35(5): 346–52.

Appendix

Appendix 1: Glossary and Abbreviations

Glossary	
Air bronchogram	Air within bronchi seen within a consolidation.
Airspace	Densities that appear fluffy (like clouds) that are indicative of consolidation.
Atelectasis	A lung process that results in volume loss. There are various patterns and types described in the Airway pattern section of this Guide.
Consolidation	Air space opacities that are fluffy (like cumulous clouds) that often indicate pneumonia. This is described in more detail in the lung parenchyma chapter.
Conspicuity	Degree of "conspicuousness." High conspicuity is an obvious finding, and a decreased conspicuity is a subtle finding. Various properties or adjacent structures may alter conspicuity.
Cysts (holes)	Fine lucencies in the lungs indicating long-term or end-stage lung disease, as described in the interstitial pattern section of this Guide.
Density	Whiteness, or any area of whiteness, on an image (opacity). Bones are an example. Imaging densities also include soft tissues (including, blood/fluid, fat, calcium, and even air low density).
Horizontal beam	When the x-ray tube is horizontally oriented relative to the patient and the x-ray beam is parallel to the floor. This is the only way to effectively demonstrate a fluid level.
Infiltrate	A non-descript term that is often used to indicate an opacity exists that may represent a consolidation, interstitial pattern, or atelectasis. From the radiologist to the provider, there is flexibility in interpretation.
Interstitial	Used to describe linear opacities that are not vessels; rather may cross vessels at angles not in branching patterns. This is described in more detail in the lung parenchyma chapter.
Edge	Any visible demarcation between a density on one side and lucency on the other.

L.R. Folio, *Chest Imaging*, DOI 10.1007/978-1-4614-1317-2_1,
© Henry M. Jackson Foundation for the Advancement of Military Medicine, Inc. 2012

Glossary	
Line	A thin density with lucency on both sides or a thin lucency with density on both sides.
Lucency	Blackness, or any area of blackness, on an image. The trachea is an example.
Mach (not mock) bands (or effect)	Center-surround receptive field interactions resulting in apparent lucencies. These often occur adjacent to curved densities next to relative lucencies (such as the right atrial heart shadow).
Nodules	Fine, well-rounded opacities that are larger than vessels on end (relatively speaking from a peripheral perspective), indicating an interstitial pattern, specifically dots.
Obliterated	Obscured structure that should otherwise be seen. Other words that can be used include masked, not seen, or not well discerned.
Projection	The path of the x-ray beam; can be a frontal projection (either PA or AP), lateral, or upright (erect), etc.
Reticulations (lines)	Linear opacities in the lungs that crisscross vessels (helping differentiate them from vessels) indicating a linear interstitial pattern should be considered.
Shadow	Anything visible on an image; hence, any specific density or lucency.
Silhouette	Synonym for edge. The loss of an edge constitutes the "silhouette sign" which occurs by adjacent structures masking out, e.g., RML consolidate obliterating right atrial edge.
Stripe	Either an edge or a line.
Summation shadow	Anatomic noise of overlapping structures. This often happens with posterior ribs overlapping vessels and anterior ribs, mimicking an infiltrate.
Tram track	Two fine parallel densities; essentially parallel lines simulating train or tram tracks indicating inflammation of bronchi, hence under airway pattern.

Abbreviations	
ARDS	Acute (or Adult) Respiratory Distress Syndrome
AP	Anterior-posterior
AVM	Arteriovenous malformation
BAC	Bronchoalveolar cell carcinoma
CIDA	Chest imaging diagnostic algorithm
COPD	Chronic obstructive pulmonary disease
CXR	Chest X-ray
CPA	Costophrenic angles
Dz	Disease
EG	Eosinophilic granuloma
ER	Emergency room
FHX	Family history
HP	Hypersensitivity pneumonitis
ICU	Intensive care unit
IVC	Inferior vena cava
LCG	Langerhans granulomatosis
LCH	Langerhans cell histiocytosis

Abbreviations	
LIP	Lymphocytic interstitial pneumonia
LPA	Left pulmonary artery
LLL	Left lower lobe
LUL	Left upper lobe
MAI	Mycobacterium avium-intracellular
MSK	Musculoskeletal
PA	Posterior-anterior
RLL	Right lower lobe
RML	Right middle lobe
RUL	Right upper lobe
RPA	Right pulmonary artery
SPN	Solitary pulmonary nodule
TB	Tuberculosis
SVC	Superior vena cava
USU	Uniformed Services University

Appendix 2: Sources and Additional References

Text Sources

Unless otherwise noted, the material within was compiled by Dr. Les Folio or borrowed from material he delivered in his lectures at Uniformed Services University.

The following sources were consulted and have been cited in the pages of this book.

ARDS secondary to hepatorenal syndrome. In: MedPix. Retrieved on September 15, 2008 from http://rad.usuhs.edu/medpix/master.php3?mode=print_case&pt_id=5117&showall=yes.

Broussard E. Pulmonary artery hypertension – shunt vascularity. In: MedPix. 2003. Retrieved on September 15, 2008 from http://rad.usuhs.edu/medpix/radpix.html?mode=single&recnum=4854&table=&srchstr=&search.

Dubois D. Miliary nodular INTERSTITIAL pattern (lung). In: Medpix. 2000. Retrieved on September 15, 2008 from http://rad.usuhs.edu/medpix/master.php3?mode=single&recnum=841&table=card&srchstr=interstitial&search=interstitial#top.

Folio LR. A mnemonic approach to the evaluation of chest x-ray films. J Am Osteopath Assoc. 1995;95(11):648.

Folio L, Feigin DS, Singleton B, Arner D. Chest imaging diagnostic assistant. Poster presented at Association of University Radiologists. Austin, TX 2006.

Folio L, Feigin D, Smirniotopoulos J, Singleton B. Chest imaging portal: educational phase. RSNA InfoRad. Chicago, IL 2006.

MacMahon H, Austin JHM, Gamsu G, Herold CJ, Jett JR, Naidich DP, Patz Jr EF, Swensen SJ. Guidelines for management of small pulmonary nodules detected on CT scans: a statement from the Fleischner Society. Radiology. 2005; 237:395–400.

National Heart Lung and Blood Institute. What is pulmonary arterial hypertension? Retrieved on 9/15/08, from http://www.nhlbi.nih.gov/health/dci/Diseases/pah/pah_what.html.

Shaffer K. Role of radiology for imaging and biopsy of solitary pulmonary nodules. Chest. 1999;116:519–22. Retrieved on October 14, 2008 from http://www.chestjournal.org/cgi/reprint/116/suppl_3/519S.pdf.

Shogan P, Muncy T, McCarthy K, Folio L. Pneumocystis jiroveci pneumonia. Mil Med Int J AMSUS. 2008;173(10):vii, viii.

Slotto J, Folio L. Cystic fibrosis chest x-ray findings: a teaching analog. Mil Med Int J AMSUS. 2008;173(7):xii, xiii.

Trask S. Hydropneumothorax. In: MedPix. 2007. Retrieved on October 16, 2008 from http://rad.usuhs.edu/medpix/medpix_home.html?mode=single&recnum=7558&table=card&srchstr=hydropneumothorax&search=hydropneumothorax#top.

Warnock A, Gibson M, Folio L. Chondroblastoma with secondary aneurysmal bone cyst. Mil Med Int J AMSUS. 2008;173(2):xiii–xiv.

Wikipedia. Pneumoconiosis. Retrieved on August 15, 2008 from http://en.wikipedia.org/wiki/Pneumoconiosis.

Yamamoto M, Kurano M, Ogawa R, Fukuoka H, Kawashima H, Ohmatsu H, Moriyama N. Quantitative evaluation method for lung tumor with fractal analysis of x-ray CT images. Annual Report of the National Institute of Radiological Sciences, Japan. 1998–1999. Retrieved May 11, 2007 from http://www.nirs.go.jp/report/nene/H10/1/003.html.

Zylak CM, Standen JR, Barnes GR, Zylak CJ. Pneumomediastinum revisited. Radiographics. 2000;20(4):1043–57.

Image Sources

Unless otherwise noted, all medical images (CXRs and CTs) are from the teaching files of the Department of Radiology & Radiological Sciences at the Uniformed Services University of the Health Sciences.

Images that were not created by the ETI Support Office are images that have been released to the public domain by their creators. The following is a list of the sources of those images.

Alveoli image on Home > Abnormal Lung Parenchyma > Consolidative: Image source: Wikipedia. Retrieved on September 16, 2008, from http://en.wikipedia.org/wiki/Alveoli.

End-stagehoneycomblungdiseaseonHome > AbnormalLungParenchyma > Interstitial: Image Source: Wikipedia. Retrieved on September 15, 2008 from http://commons.wikimedia.org/wiki/Image:End-stage_interstitial_lung_disease_(honeycomb_lung).jpg.

Face-vase illusion on Home > Abnormal Lung Parenchyma > Consolidative > Consolidative Model: Image source: Wikipedia. Retrieved on October 22, 2008 from http:///wiki/Image:en.wikipedia.orgMultistability.jpg.

Additional References

Chest Imaging References

Slotto J, Folio L. Cystic fibrosis chest x-ray findings: a teaching analog. Mil Med Int J AMSUS. 2008;173(7):xii, xiii.

Warnock A, Gibson M, Folio L. Chondroblastoma with secondary aneurysmal bone cyst. Mil Med Int J AMSUS. 2008;173(2):xiii–xiv.

Shogan P, Muncy T, McCarthy K, Folio L. Pneumocystis jiroveci pneumonia. Mil Med Int J AMSUS. 2008;173(10):vii–viii.

Folio LR. A mnemonic approach to the evaluation of chest x-ray films. J Am Osteopath Assoc. 1995;95(11):648.

Chest Imaging Online References

Folio L. Chest review portal. http://rad.usuhs.edu/medpix/topic_display.html?mode= single&recnum=6043#top. Accessed 26 May 2011.

Carpenter W. Basic chest x-ray review. http://rad.usuhs.mil/rad/chest_review/ index.html. Accessed 26 May 2011.

Folio L, Feigin D, Smirniotopoulos J. Basic chest imaging review, search pattern, required structures. In: MedPix. 2007. http://rad.usuhs.edu/medpix/topic_display.ht ml?mode=single&recnum=6043#top. Accessed 26 May 2011.

Feigin D. Case studies (takes you through several abnormal CXRs to test your search pattern and recognition skills). http://rad.usuhs.mil/rad/handouts/feigin/ abnlcxr/myindex.htm. Accessed 26 May 2011.

Chestreview–popupanatomy.http://rad.usuhs.mil/medpix/medpix.html?mode=pt&pt_ id=6204&quiz=no&imid=17678#top. Accessed 26 May 2011.

Webb D. HRCT chest primer. http://pathhsw5m54.ucsf.edu/ctpath/ctpathcontents. html. Accessed 26 May 2011.

MS 2 final exam example questions used in the past. http://rad.usuhs.mil/medpix/ medpix.html?mode=exam_review&exam=131#top. Accessed 26 May 2011.

LearningRadiology.com. http://www.learningradiology.com/medstudents/22mu stsformedstudents_files/v3_document.htm. Accessed 26 May 2011.

MS-2 radiologic interpretation course. http://rad.usuhs.mil/rad/handouts/ms-2_ final.html. Accessed 26 May 2011.

Index

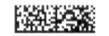